SMALL *Oxford* BOOKS

DOCTORS & PATIENTS

SMALL *Oxford* BOOKS

❀❧❀

DOCTORS & PATIENTS

❀❧❀

Compiled by
DANNIE ABSE

Oxford New York
OXFORD UNIVERSITY PRESS
1984

Oxford University Press, Walton Street, Oxford OX2 6DP

London New York Toronto
Delhi Bombay Calcutta Madras Karachi
Kuala Lumpur Singapore Hong Kong Tokyo
Nairobi Dar es Salaam Cape Town
Melbourne Auckland

and associated companies in
Beirut Berlin Ibadan Mexico City Nicosia

Oxford is a trade mark of Oxford University Press

British Library Cataloguing in Publication Data

Doctors and patients.—(Small Oxford books)
1. Medicine in literature
I. Abse, Dannie
808.8'0356 PN6071.M38
ISBN 0-19-214148-1

Library of Congress Cataloging in Publication Data

Main entry under title:
Doctors & patients.
(Small Oxford books)
Includes index.
1. Medicine—Miscellanea. I. Abse, Dannie.
II. Title: Doctors and patients.
R706.D63 1984 610 83-24998
ISBN 0-19-214148-1

Set by Grove Graphics
Printed in Great Britain by
Hazell Watson & Viney Limited
Aylesbury, Bucks

Introduction

It would seem we are inexhaustibly intrigued by the figure of the doctor and it is not only because, sooner or later, we all become patients. The doctor is a confidence man, not necessarily in the worst sense. He is rarely depicted neutrally, whether on the page or in the theatre, or on the screen: he is either charismatic healer, idealized hero to be revered; or a demonic figure to be distrusted; or simply a buffoon to be mocked. In short, however sceptical or sophisticated we imagine ourselves to be we are somewhat in awe of him, especially at three o'clock in the morning when a light may be on in one particular bedroom upstairs.

And is not the very act of *persistent* mockery of the doctor, so wonderfully performed, say, by a Molière or a Shaw, or in long centuries past by one such as Pliny, who complained that the Greek physician was the only citizen who could kill another with sovereign impunity, proof of more than a vestigial awe? Their mockery, justified and moral and doubtless socially useful, also allowed their own unacknowledged awe to be deflated and tamed.

Something primitive in us, deep down, surely leads us to half-fancy that there are secrets in this world that some men are privy to – secrets antecedent to all recorded history and, in more recent times, translated into Latin and Greek from the hieroglyphs of a lost language. These secrets some doctors, perhaps, have in their possession – and if we know that this is not so when we are healthy, we may well think otherwise when we are stressfully ill. Then, longing for a wizard, we send for his surrogate, the doctor, who bears no wand but a stethoscope and a prescription.

Oliver Sacks is surely right when he declares, 'There is, of course, an ordinary medicine, an everyday medicine, humdrum, prosaic, a medicine for stubbed toes, quinsies, bunions and boils; but all of us entertain the idea of *another* sort of medicine of a wholly different kind: something deeper, older, extraordinary, almost sacred, which will restore us our lost health and wholeness.' That other medicine is one of the secrets.

As a doctor myself I say to you, the reader — patient or fellow physician, hospital visitor or nurse — that there is another secret in this little book. I say it with confidence though I am not sure whether or not I'm joking.

Will you find it? Should you quest for it, and I hope you will, it will be my fault if, in so doing, you are not sometimes arrested by the drama of facts, amused by the absurdity of the human predicament, and sometimes, too, moved by the pity of it all.

D. A.

Ogmore-by-Sea, 1983

At Medical School

Everything in Yura's mind was mixed up together and misplaced and everything was sharply his own — his views, his habits and his inclinations. He was unusually impressionable and the freshness and novelty of his vision were remarkable.

Though he was greatly drawn to art and history, he scarcely hesitated over the choice of his career. He considered that art was no more a vocation than innate cheerfulness or melancholy were professions. He was interested in physics and natural science and believed that a man should do something useful in his practical life. He settled on medicine.

In the first year of his four-year course he had spent a term in the dissecting room; it was deep underground in the basement of the university. You came down the winding staircase. There was always a crowd of dishevelled students, some hard at work over their tattered textbooks surrounded by bones, or quietly dissecting, each in his corner, others fooling about, cracking jokes and chasing the rats which scurried in swarms over the stone floors. In the half-darkness of the mortuary the naked bodies of drowned women and unidentified young suicides, well preserved and untouched by decay, gleamed white as phosphorus. Injections of alum salts rejuvenated them and gave them a deceptive roundness. The corpses were cut open, dismembered and prepared, yet even in its smallest sections the human body kept its beauty, so that the wonder Yura felt in looking at the body of a young girl brutally flung down upon a zinc table he also felt in gazing at her amputated arm or hand. The basement smelled of carbolic and formaldehyde and was filled with the presence of mystery, the mystery of the unknown lives of these naked dead, and the mystery of life and death itself — and death was as familiar in this place as though the underground room were its home or its headquarters.

The voice of this mystery, drowning everything else, distracted Yura at his dissecting. But then a lot of things in life distracted him. He was used to it and was not put out.

Boris Pasternak, *Doctor Zhivago*, 1958

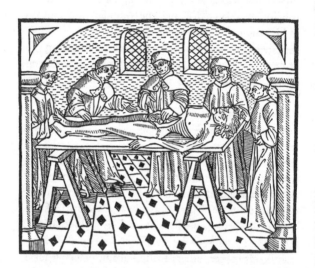

Become a doctor! Study anatomy! Dissect! Witness horrible operations instead of throwing myself heart and soul into the glorious art of music! Forsake the empyrean for the dreary realities of earth! The immortal angels of poetry and love and their inspired songs for filthy hospitals, dreadful medical students, hideous corpses, the shriek of patients, the groans and death rattles of the dying. It seemed to be the utter reversal of the natural conditions of my life — horrible and impossible. Yet it came to pass.

Hector Berlioz, *Memoirs*, 1870

From the outset of their apprenticeship some medical students do not seem fitted to become, one day, respon-

[2]

*sible physicians or surgeons. Hector Berlioz, always
more interested in music than medicine, was one such:*

On arriving in Paris in 1822 with my fellow-student
Alphonse Robert, I gave myself up wholly to studying
for the career which had been thrust upon me, and
loyally kept the promise I had given my father on
leaving. It was soon put to a somewhat severe test when
Robert, having announced one morning that he had
bought a 'subject' (a corpse) took me for the first time
to the dissecting-room at the Hospice de la Pitié. At
the sight of that terrible charnel-house — the fragments
of limbs, the grinning heads and gaping skulls, the
bloody quagmire underfoot and the atrocious smell it
gave off, the swarms of sparrows wrangling over scraps
of lung, the rats in their corner gnawing the bleeding
vertebrae — such a feeling of revulsion possessed me
that I leapt through the window of the dissecting-room
and fled for home as though Death and all his hideous
train were at my heels. The shock of that first impression lasted for about twenty-four hours. I did not want
to hear another word about anatomy, dissection or
medicine, and I meditated a hundred mad schemes of
escape from the future that hung over me.

Robert lavished his eloquence in a vain attempt to
argue away my disgust and demonstrate the absurdity
of my plans. In the end he got me to agree to make
another effort. For the second time I accompanied him
to the hospital and we entered the house of the dead.
How strange! The objects which before had filled me
with extreme horror had absolutely no effect upon me
now. I felt nothing but a cold distaste; I was already
as hardened to the scene as any seasoned medical
student. The crisis was past. I found I actually enjoyed
groping about in a poor fellow's chest and feeding the
winged inhabitants of that delightful place their ration
of lung. 'Hallo!' Robert cried, laughing, 'you're getting
civilized. Giving the birds their meat in due season.'
'And filling all things living with plenteousness,' I

retorted, tossing a shoulder-blade to a great rat that was staring at me with famished eyes.

So I went on with my anatomy course, feeling no enthusiasm, but stoically resigned.

Hector Berlioz, *Memoirs*, 1870

Did Berlioz ever wonder about the owner of that shoulder-blade? There was, at that time, a thriving trade in body-snatching. In Britain, a corpse would fetch between seven and twelve guineas from the medical schools — plus expenses! No surprise, therefore, that cemeteries were burgled and cadavers delivered to the anatomy students for dissection. Even more distressing, people were murdered for this purpose.

A fearful excitement had been created in all parts of the country by stories of murders committed and graves robbed of their ghastly tenants for the purpose of supplying with 'subjects' the dissecting tables of the London and Edinburgh schools of anatomy. In the latter city two miscreants named Burke and Hare had been convicted of murder and one of them hanged for their crimes; but the scare had not abated. Stories were told with appalling frequency of corpses missing from lonely graveyards and of narrow escapes from murder in little-frequented places. As the dark nights of the late autumn came on, the fears of the timid and nervous were doubled, and persons who lived in lonely places, or in the ill-lighted parts of towns, became afraid to leave their houses after nightfall. I remember hearing such fears expressed by several persons at Croydon with whom my parents were acquainted, and also of neighbours combining to assist in watching the graves of deceased members of each others' families.

Burkers and Body-Snatchers, 1876

'Twas in the middle of the night,
To sleep young William tried
When Mary's Ghost came stealing in
And stood at his bedside.

O William dear! O William dear!
My rest eternal ceases:
Alas my everlasting peace
Is broken into pieces.

The body-snatchers they have come,
And made a snatch at me.
It's very hard them kind of men
Won't let a body be!

The arm that used to take your arm
Is took to Dr Vyse
And both my legs are going to walk
The hospital at Guy's.

I vowed you would have my hand
But fate gives me denial;
You'll find it there at Dr Bell's
In spirits and a phial.

The cock it crows; I must be gone
My William, we must part;
Though I'll be yours in death,
Sir Astley has my heart.

Thomas Hood (1799–1845), 'Mary's Ghost'

In the foyer of a great medical school there hangs a painting of Vesalius. Lean, ascetic, possessed, the anatomist stands before a dissecting table upon which lies the naked body of a man. The flesh of the two is silvery. A concentration of moonlight, like a strange rain of virus, washes them. The cadaver has dignity and reserve; it is distanced by its death. Vesalius reaches for his dissecting knife. As he does so, he glances over his shoulder at a crucifix on the wall. His face wears an expression of guilt and melancholy and fear. He knows that there is something wrong, forbidden in what he is about to do, but he cannot help himself, for he is a fanatic. He is driven by a dark desire. To see, to feel, to discover is all. His is a passion, not a romance.

I understand you, Vesalius. Even now, after so many voyages within, so much exploration, I feel the same sense that one must not gaze into the body, the same irrational fear that it is an evil deed for which punishment awaits. Consider. The sight of our internal organs is denied us. To how many men is it given to look upon their own spleens, their hearts, and live? The hidden geography of the body is a Medusa's head one glimpse of which would render blind the presumptuous eye. Still, rigid rules are broken by the smallest inadvertencies: I pause in the midst of an operation being performed under spinal anaesthesia to observe the face of my patient, to speak a word or two of reassurance. I peer above the screen separating his head from his abdomen, in which I am most deeply employed. He is not asleep, but rather stares straight upward, his attention riveted, a look of terrible discovery, of wonder upon his face. Watch him. This man is violating a taboo. I follow his gaze upward, and see in the great operating lamp suspended above his belly the reflection of his viscera. There is the liver, dark and turgid above, there the loops of his bowel winding slow, there his blood runs extravagantly. It is that which he sees and studies with so much horror and fascination. Something primordial in him has been aroused — a fright, a longing. I feel it, too, and quickly bend above his open body to shield it from his view. How dare he look within the Ark! Cover his eyes! But it is too late; he has already *seen*; that which no man should; he has trespassed. And I am no longer a surgeon, but a hierophant who must do magic to ward off the punishment of the angry gods.

Richard Selzer, *Mortal Lessons*, 1974

In 1957 the late Lord Platt was elected President of the Royal College of Physicians. When a student, like Berlioz he found the dissecting-room distasteful and, as a result, sometimes neglected his studies; he played the piano instead. Unlike Berlioz, however, he was 'a born

doctor' as this account of his First Consultation in a
Sheffield boarding-house suggests.

My landlady at that time was an attractive and passionate foreign woman who was ill-assorted with her
rather vulgar husband, and much more attached to one
of her lodgers. One day, when I was practising on her
grand piano, and cutting my lectures and attendances
at the women's hospital, she came into the room to
ask my advice. She wanted to discuss with me various
ways in which she could murder her husband. I
remember the occasion as a factual conversation without any obvious show of emotion. I rapidly realized
that I might be deemed an accessory if I gave her any
good advice and confined my attention to telling her
the various ways in which her plans could be found
out. I prize that memory as being My First Consultation. My Second Consultation was when her lover
(back from the War) knocked her husband out and
came to seek my opinion as to whether he was dead.
Fortunately (for me at any rate) he was only concussed
and already showing signs of recovery before I arrived
on the scene. There must be few, if any physicians
whose first consultations were so challenging. Perhaps
they were a good preparation for the life to come. At
least I learnt the need for calm deliberation and self-
control.

Lord Platt in *My Medical School*, 1978

Of course the dissecting-room in Lord Platt's day —
during the First World War — was not as horrific as
that which Hector Berlioz encountered. Certainly it
was not so later, by the time of the Second World
War when I began my medical studies. Yet dissecting
a corpse still seemed to me then a dolorous enough
exercise.

Most of the time we, too, investigated that forlorn
thing, the cadaver and pried into its bloodless meat that
had pickling formaldehyde in its arteries. The sour

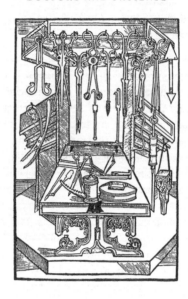

formaldehyde fumes would stay with us, soak into our very clothes. Still we dug into the material of dead flesh with scalpel — scraped it, stripped it, cut deep into it, learned its thoroughways, yet had no spiritual shock of revelation. Our first disgust weakened to distaste and our distaste was usurped by numbness, by an apathetic neutrality.

This progression of feelings arriving at non-feeling was true, I think, for even the most sensitive student. For the neck, say, exposed with all its muscles and its vessels mimicking a coloured plate in the anatomy book, seemed, soon enough, never to have belonged to a live person. The wonder of a hand, say, provoked no abstract questions, even in our youthful minds, about God or Death or the Meaning of Life — no metaphysical speculation whatsoever. That was to come later when we 'walked the wards' in hospital and attended post-mortems of people we had spoken to a day earlier. But now this hand, or rather this resemblance of a hand, had never held, it seemed, another hand in greeting or in tenderness, had never clenched a fist in anger, had never held a pen to sign an authentic name. For this thing, this — as the weeks, the months, passed by — decreasing thing, visibly losing its 'divine proportions', this residue, this so-called trunk of a body, this legless, armless, headless thing had never had a name surely?

Dannie Abse, A *Poet in the Family*, 1974

My first consultation as a medical student, like that of Lord Platt, was also somewhat bizarre. My eldest brother had given me a letter of introduction to his friend, the Westminster Hospital psychiatrist, Dr Ewing. So, one afternoon, I attended Psychiatric Out-patients.

That afternoon another psychiatrist was taking Out-patients. He had a strong Viennese accent, a most reassuring thing in a psychiatrist, and he seemed pleased to see me. In fact he was enthusiastic. 'You can take Out-patients yourself,' he beamed. 'You've come just in time.' Startled, I explained that I had only been at Westminster Hospital three weeks or so and did not feel capable of taking on any out-patients, never mind psychiatric ones. 'I haf to be somevere at three,' he said. 'It is good. And don't vorry, you know how to take a case history, yes? Zen take a case history and tell them to return next week ven I vill see them myself.' Even as I was objecting he was racing for the door shouting, 'Nurse! Nurse!'

So, wearing a white coat, I sat behind a desk like a real doctor and the nurse sent in the first patient for me to see. My very own first patient. I knew how to take a case history. Only a week earlier I had been taught that in Casualty. First you had to put down *Complaining of*, and then you asked the patient, 'What are you complaining of?' and the patient would say, 'I have a pain in my left chest, doctor, that comes on after exercise.' And so you would write that down opposite *Complaining of*. It was quite simple really. Then there were other headings such as *Past History*,

Present History, and so on. Easy as winking. Except my first patient complained of his wife. 'She gets up in the middle of the night,' he told me, 'because she reckons she hears voices. Then she walks up and down, walks up and down for hours and hours. I can't stand it.' After listening to his grumbles, inspired I said, 'Now I want you to bring your wife here next week and then we'll sort things out.' To my horror he replied, 'But she's outside, doctor. She's come along with me.' It was evident that I had to see her so, swallowing, I nodded and said, 'Then I'll see her right away. Would you mind waiting outside?'

His wife baffled me. She complained of her husband. 'He says he hears voices and gets up in the middle of the night and walks up and down remorselessly for hours. I can't bear it,' she said.

I did not know which one was crazy, who was hallucinating, which one was telling the truth. On her case-history sheet I wrote 'complaining of her husband's strange insomnia' and on his case-history sheet I wrote 'complaining of his wife's strange insomnia'. And the following week I never came back when they came back and I avoided that Viennese doctor ever after. The great thing was they both had called me 'doctor'. Neither of them called me 'sonny'.

Dannie Abse, A *Strong Dose of Myself*, 1983

But what of the teachers of medical students? Baglivi has said, 'The patient is the doctor's best text-book.' That 'text-book' however has to be introduced to the student and those who effect the introductions are not always wise. Few, though, could be as ignorant as Keats's surgeon-teacher, Billy Lucas, who practised surgery without ever learning anatomy! Keats, by the way, registered as Lucas's dresser, or assistant, on 3 March 1816.

In the front three rows with the other dressers and apprentices, he could see everything that went on at close quarters. It was not only the groans of the patient, half-stupefied with rum, or, worse, the cries of the children that could shake one; worst of all was the terrifying lack of skill of some of the surgeons. At this point, luck or influence deserted Keats. Instead of the temporary dressership under Astley Cooper, which Henry Cooper had held and in which Keats had perhaps deputized, he was now appointed to the dressership left vacant by William Bentham Everest under William Lucas, junior, the son of Hammond's master. Dogged by ill-health, including premature deafness, 'Billy' Lucas had never been fit enough to study anatomy in the unhealthy dissecting-room of his day; but the influence of a successful father proved stronger than this handicap, and in 1799 he duly succeeded to the parental position as surgeon in the hospital. Here he began a career of butchery which even his generous colleague, Astley Cooper, was to recall with critical horror: 'he was neat-handed, but rash in the extreme, cutting amongst most important parts as though they were only skin, and making us all shudder from apprehension of his opening arteries or committing some other error'. He put students off surgery not, as has been suggested, because he was dull, but because he was dangerous; the person most to appreciate the danger was his own dresser, left to clear up the mess he had made.

Robert Gittings, *John Keats*, 1968

*Worse, in those days no anaesthetics were available —
nitrous oxide (laughing-gas) and ether were not discovered until 1842–7. And the only means to reduce
operative pain was through soporifics — opium, hemp,
hashish, and whisky.*

In a case of amputation, it was the custom to bring the patient into the operating room and place him upon the table. The surgeon would stand with his hands behind his back and would say to the patient, 'Will you have your leg off, or will you not have it off?' If the patient lost courage and said, no, he had decided not to have the leg amputated, he was at once carried back to his bed in the ward. If, however, he said, 'Yes' he was immediately taken firmly in hand by a number of strong assistants and the operation went on regardless of whatever he might say thereafter. If his courage failed him *after* this crucial moment, it was too late and no attention was paid to his cries of protest. It was found to be the only practicable method by which an operation could be performed under the gruesome conditions which prevailed before the advent of anaesthesia.

J. Collins Warren, *To Work in the Vineyard of Surgery*, 1958

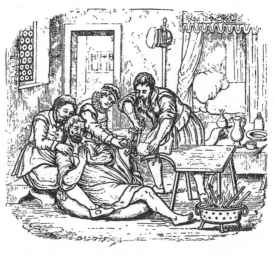

The medical student was thus exposed to brutal experiences very early on in his career. Moreover, he had to pay for it dearly, especially in the USA.

Very well do I remember the first Monday in November 1830. I then entered the Medical School in Cincinnati as a student. All of the professors, that morning, at nine o'clock, were sitting around a long, wide table. Commencing at one, paying fees and taking tickets, every student continued until he had made the entire round. To the best of my recollection, each professor, that morning, got about six hundred dollars.

Quoted in Otto Juettner's *Daniel Drake and his Followers*, 1909

Among the present-day teachers of medical students there may be no butchering Billy Lucas. But some must be judged as very rum indeed:

Of Barcroft there are, of course, numerous anecdotes. Like Haldane, he was interested in the role of haemoglobin, and he became interested in the spleen at a time when little or nothing was known of its functions. It is said that he once asked a somewhat frightened candidate to tell him what were the functions of the spleen. After a few moments of panic the student blurted out, 'I'm afraid, sir, I've forgotten.' 'Good Lord,' said Barcroft, 'now *nobody* knows.' Later, when he had become interested in the spleen's possible role as a regulator of the volume of circulating blood, he came to Sheffield to lecture on 'The Spleen' to the Medico-Chirurgical Society. He started with the somewhat unexpected words, 'Ladies and Gentlemen, with the exception of the penis, the spleen alters its size more than any other organ of the body.'

Lord Platt in *My Medical School*, 1978

There was no briefing for the neophyte, nothing resembling our present introductory courses. One plunged straight in. My first lecture in the adjacent medical school was by coincidence given by the oculist I was destined to succeed, A. F. MacCallan, and he opened it by displaying on our old epidiascope the frontispiece of the book he had written on Trachoma, showing a bust of himself, in glory outside the hospital in Cairo that he had founded. Some weeks later Sir Stanley Woodward opened his lecture by producing a gold 'demi-hunter' watch from his waistcoat pocket, declaring that this was the first requisite for a doctor, since it inspired confidence; the rest of his lecture discussed the virtues of the different European spas.

After this lecture came the ward-round. I had been allocated to the firm of our then Senior Physician, Hildred Carlill, a quasi-neurologist, who practised rather elementary hypnosis on many of his patients, in the main quite successfully, although often for bizarre reasons (Now repeat, 'I must not have intercourse with my wife while she is pregnant'; now once again 'I must not . . .'); he also, like Shaw's Cutler Walpole, firmly believed in the 'nuciform sac' as the cause of most ills (if he inserted his long forefinger, and pressed hard into the right pelvis, he could nearly always elicit some appendicular tenderness). It was a formidable start to clinical medicine, but not very arduous since a third of our patients were spending weeks under Somnifane narcosis (hoping to remedy their habit-spasms and so on), and another third were mourning the loss of their (apparently sound) appendices. Carlill, I soon discovered, had more idiosyncrasies than most of his fellow consultants, to whom he was often rather an embarrassment. Indeed, on one occasion he was sued by a female patient, whose limp he reckoned was hysterical, for forcing her to demonstrate her gait, stripped to the panties, in front of the boardroom. But in those days, high-handed eccentricities were expected of the more senior consultants who, since they were unpaid for their services, were very hard to discipline or control. Indeed, Carlill's predecessor, Sir James Purves-Stewart, was even less inhibited: he processed through his wards like a bishop followed by his house-surgeon bearing a gold patella hammer, then a secretary ready to record his comments, then his chauffeur carrying the box of other instruments, and then his disciples. At the end of his career he proclaimed that he had found a vaccine for multiple sclerosis, and the queue of wretched sufferers stretched daily into the abbey sanctuary, waiting for the miracle cure. When the treatment was exposed, Sir James retired to the safe isolation of a

lighthouse on the Sussex Coast, and was never seen
again at Westminster.

Patrick Trevor-Roper in *My Medical School*, 1978

*After years of spiritual trauma, cramming, and minor
enlightenment, the medical student takes his qualifying
examinations and, if successful, is let loose on the
world; but the ordeal of an oral examination in particular hasn't changed that much over the last two
hundred years — as can be seen from Smollett's*
Roderick Random.

A young fellow came out from the place of examination with a pale countenance, his lip quivering, and his
looks as wild as if he had seen a ghost. He no sooner
appeared, than we all flocked about him with the
utmost eagerness to know what reception he had met
with; which, after some pause, he described, recounting
all the questions they had asked, with the answers he
made. In this manner, we obliged no less than twelve
to recapitulate, which, now the danger was past, they
did with pleasure, before it fell to my lot: at length
the beadle called my name, with a voice that made me
tremble as much as if it had been the sound of the
last trumpet: however there was no remedy: I was conducted into a large hall, where I saw about a dozen
of grim faces sitting at a long table; one of whom bade
me come forward, in such an imperious tone that I
was actually for a minute or two bereft of my senses.
The first question he put to me was, 'Where was you
born?' To which I answered, 'In Scotland.' 'In Scotland,' said he; 'I know that very well; we have scarce
any other countrymen to examine here; you Scotchmen
have overspread us of late as the locusts did Egypt: I
ask you in what part of Scotland was you born?' I
named the place of my nativity, which he had never
before heard of: he then proceeded to interrogate me
about my age, the town where I served my time, with
the term of my apprenticeship; and when I informed

him that I served three years only, he fell into a violent passion; swore it was a shame and a scandal to send such raw boys into the world as surgeons; that it was a great presumption in me, and an affront upon the English, to pretend to sufficient skill in my business, having served so short a time, when every apprentice in England was bound seven years at least; that my friends would have done better if they had made me a weaver or shoemaker, but their pride would have me a gentleman, he supposed, at any rate, and their poverty could not afford the necessary education.

This exordium did not at all contribute to the recovery of my spirits, but, on the contrary reduced me to such a situation that I was scarce able to stand; which being perceived by a plump gentleman who sat opposite to me, with a skull before him, he said, Mr Snarler was too severe upon the young man; and, turning towards me, told me, I need not to be afraid, for nobody would do me any harm; then bidding me take time to recollect myself, he examined me touching the operation of the trepan, and was very well satisfied with my answers. The next person who questioned me was a wag, who began by asking if I had ever seen amputation performed; and I replying in the affirmative, he shook his head, and said, 'What! upon a dead subject, I suppose?' 'If,' continued he, 'during an engagement at sea, a man should be brought to you with his head shot off, how would you behave?' After some hesitation I owned such a case had never come under my observation, neither did I remember to have seen any method of cure proposed for such an accident, in any of the systems of surgery I had perused. Whether it was owing to the simplicity of my answer, or the archness of the question, I know not, but every member of the board deigned to smile, except Mr Snarler, who seemed to have very little of the *animal risibile* in his constitution.

Tobias Smollett, *The Adventures of Roderick Random*, 1748

Today when a student finally qualifies as a doctor he is given a glass of sherry by his examiners, asked solemnly to sign a document, and in a kind of dazed euphoria, swears to abide by the spirit of the age-old Hippocratic oath.

I swear by Apollo the healer, and Asclepius, and Hygeia, and All-heal (Panacea) and all the gods and goddesses . . . that, according to my ability and judgement, I will keep this Oath and this stipulation — to reckon him who taught me this Art as dear to me as those who bore me . . . to look upon his offspring as my own brothers, and to teach them this Art, if they would learn it, without fee or stipulation. By precept, lecture, and all other modes of instruction, I will impart a knowledge of the Art to my own sons, and those of my teacher, and to disciples bound by a stipulation and oath according to the Law of Medicine, but to none other. I will follow that system of regimen which, according to my ability and judgement, I consider for the benefit of my patients, and abstain from whatever is deleterious and mischievous. I will give no deadly medicine to anyone if asked, nor suggest any such counsel; nor will I aid a woman to produce abortion. With purity and holiness I will pass my life and practise my Art. . . Into whatever houses I enter, I will go there for the benefit of the sick, and will abstain from every act of mischief and corruption; and above all from seduction. . . Whatever in my professional practice — or even not in connection with it — I see and hear in the lives of men which ought not to be spoken of abroad, I will not divulge, deeming that on such matters we should be silent. While I keep this Oath unviolated, may it be granted me to enjoy life and the practice of the Art, always respected among men: but should I break or violate this Oath, may the reverse be my lot.

The Legacy of Greece, ed. R. Livingstone, 1921

Good Doctors, Bad Doctors

> Wherever a doctor cannot do good, he must be kept
> from doing harm.
>
> Hippocrates

I have heard it said that the art of healing makes men
hard-hearted and indifferent to human suffering. I am
willing to own that there is often a professional hard-
ness in surgeons, just as there is in theologians — only
much less in degree than in these last. It does not
commonly improve the sympathies of a man to be in
the habit of thrusting knives into his fellow-creatures
and burning them with red-hot irons, any more than
it improves them to hold the blinding-white cautery of
Gehenna by its cool handle and score and crisp young
souls with it until they are scorched into the belief of
Transubstantiation or the Immaculate Conception. And,
to say the plain truth, I think there are a good many
coarse people in both callings. A delicate nature will
not commonly choose a pursuit which implies the
habitual infliction of suffering, so readily as some
gentler office. Yet while I am writing this paragraph,
there passes by my window, on his daily errand of
duty, not seeing me, though I catch a glimpse of his
manly features through the oval glass of his chaise, as
he rides by, a surgeon of skill and standing, so friendly,
so modest, so tender-hearted in all his ways, that, if he
had not approved himself at once adroit and firm, one
would have said he was of too kindly a mould to be the
minister of pain, even if it were saving pain.

You may be sure that some men, even among those
who have chosen the task of pruning their fellow-
creatures, grow more and more thoughtful and compassionate in the midst of their cruel experience. They

become less nervous, but more sympathetic. They have a truer sensibility for others' pain, the more they study pain and disease in the light of science.

Oliver Wendell Holmes, *The Professor at the Breakfast-Table*, 1860

The high ideals that tenuously inspire those who practise modern medicine can be traced back to the figure and spirit of Hippocrates himself. From the eighty-seven treatises of the Hippocratic Corpus the method of Hippocrates can be understood, and some idea gained of the man. He was born of a long line of physicians, in about 460 BC on the island of Cos, and led a wandering life.

We cannot exaggerate the influence on the course of medicine and the value for physicians of all time of the traditional picture that was early formed of him and that may indeed well be drawn again from the works bearing his name. In beauty and dignity that figure is beyond praise. . . Hippocrates will ever remain the type of the perfect physician, learned, observant, humane, with a profound reverence for the claims of his patients, but an overmastering desire that his experience shall benefit others, orderly and calm, disturbed only by his anxiety to record his knowledge for the use of his brother physicians and for the relief of suffering, grave, thoughtful and reticent, pure of mind and master of his passions, this is no overdrawn picture of the Father of Medicine as he appeared to his contemporaries and successors.

Charles Singer in *The Legacy of Greece*, 1921

Hippocrates' contemporary, Plato, believed that the best doctors should have experienced disease themselves.

The most skilful physicians are those who, from their youth upwards, have combined with the knowledge of their art the greatest experience of disease; they had better not be robust in health, and should have had all manner of disease in their own persons. For the

body, as I conceive, is not the instrument with which
they cure the body; in that case we could not allow
them ever to be or to have been sickly; but they
cure the body with the mind, and the mind which has
become and is sick can cure nothing.

Plato (c.427–347 BC), *The Republic*

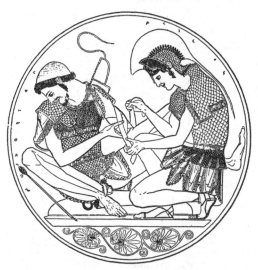

*Plato classified two types of doctors. There were those
who treated the freemen and there were those who
treated the slaves.*

Did you ever observe that there are two classes of
patients in states, slaves and freemen; and the slave
doctors run about and cure the slaves, or wait for
them in dispensaries — practitioners of this sort never
talk to their patients individually or let them talk
about their own individual complaints. The slave doctor
prescribes what mere experience suggests, as if he had
exact knowledge, and when he has given his orders,
like a tyrant, he rushes off with equal assurance to
some other servant who is ill. But the other doctor
who is a freeman, attends and practises on freemen;
and he carries his inquiries far back, and goes into the

nature of the disorder; he enters into discourse with
the patient and with his friends, and is at once getting
information from the sick man and also instructing
him as far as he is able, and he will not prescribe until
he has at first convinced him. If one of those empirical
physicians, who practise medicine without science, were
to come upon the gentleman physician talking to his
gentleman patient and using the language almost of
philosophy, beginning at the beginning of the disease
and discoursing about the whole nature of the body,
he would burst into a hearty laugh — he would say
what most of those who are called doctors always
have at their tongues' end: Foolish fellow, he would
say, you are not healing the sick man but educating
him, and he does not want to be made a doctor but
to get well.

Plato, ibid.

No doubt those who treated the freemen could some-
times earn enormous incomes, especially those who were
most successful. So it has been through the centuries.
Pliny tells us of those who made fortunes in Rome:
Thessalus and Crinas of Massilia (who used astrology
so successfully and who forbade his patients to eat or
drink except with regard to the times and the seasons,
and who in his own time and season bequeathed ten
millions) and also M. Charmis, another Massilian:

All of a sudden one M. Charmis . . . entered the city of
Rome and not only condemned the former proceedings
of the ancient Physicians but put down the baths and
hothouses. He brought in bathing in cold water and
persuaded folk to use the same even in the middle of
winter. Nay, he feared not to give direction to his sick
patients to sit in tubs of cold water. I assure you I
have myself seen ancient Senators, such as had been
Consuls of Rome, all chilling and quaking, yea and
stark again for cold, in these kind of baths; and yet
they would seem to endure the same to show how
hardy they were. There is a treatise extant by Seneca

in which he highly approves of this course. Undoubtedly such Physicians as these who won credit and estimation by such novelties and strange devices, shoot at no other mark but to make merchandise and enrich themselves with the hazard of our lives. From this come these lamentable and woeful consultations of theirs about their patients, wherein you will see them argue and disagree in opinion, while one man cannot abide another man's judgement seeming to carry away the credit of the cure. Hence arose the Epitaph of him (whoever he was) that caused these words to be graven on his unhappy tomb, *Turba medicorum perii*, that is, The variance of a sort of Physicians about me was the cause of my death.

Pliny the Elder (AD 23–79) *Historia Naturalis*

An altogether more benign physician of that time and place was Asclepiades, who aimed to please his patients in his treatment of them.

He laid down that there were only five principal remedies which served for all diseases in common; to wit, in Diet, Abstinence in meat, Forbearing wine, Rubbing of the body and the Exercise of riding on horseback or in a carriage. He so far prevailed with his eloquence that everybody gave ear and applauded his words, because they were ready enough to believe those things to be true which were easiest, and because they saw it was in everybody's power to perform what he recommended. So by this new doctrine of his he drew all the world into a singular admiration of him as of a man descended from heaven to cure their griefs and remedies. In addition to this he had a wonderful dexterity to follow men's humours and content their appetites by promising and allowing the sick to drink wine, also in giving them cold water when he saw the opportune moment, and all to gratify his patients. And just as Cleophants had the reputation among the ancients for bringing wine into favour and setting out its virtues, so Asclepiades, desirous to grow into credit and reputation by some new invention of his own, brought up the allowing of cold water to sick persons: and (as M. Varro reports) took pleasure in being called the Cold-water Physician.

He had besides other pretty devices to flatter and please his patients. At one time he would cause them to have hanging litters or beds like cradles so that by moving and rocking to and fro he might either send them to sleep or ease the pains of their sickness. At other times he ordered the use of baths, a thing he knew folk were most desirous of; and there were besides many other fine conceits very plausible in hearing and agreeable to man's nature.

One thing we Romans may well be ashamed of, that such an old fellow as he, coming out of Greece (the vainest nation under the sun) and beginning as he did from nothing, should (only to enrich himself) lead the whole world on a string and all of a sudden set down rules and orders for the health of mankind — laws, be it remembered, which have been as it were repealed and annulled by many that came after him.

Pliny the Elder, ibid.

Doctors have ever been praised or blamed, thought of as heroes or as villains, as these extracts from Chaucer and Fielding show.

With us there was a doctor, a physician;
Nowhere in all the world was one to match him
Where medicine was concerned, or surgery;
Being well grounded in astrology
He'd watch his patient with the utmost care
Until he'd found a favourable hour
By means of astrology, to give treatment.
Skilled to pick out the astrologic moment
For charms and talismans to aid the patient,
He knew the cause of every malady
If it were 'hot' or 'cold' or 'moist' or 'dry',
And where it came from, and from which humour;
He really was a fine practitioner.

Knowing the cause, and having found its root,
He'd soon give the sick man an antidote.
Ever at hand he had apothecaries
To send him syrups, drugs, and remedies,
For each put money in the other's pocket —
Theirs was no newly-founded partnership.
Well-read was he in Aesculapius,
In Dioscorides, and in Rufus,
Ancient Hippocrates, Hali, and Galen,
Avicenna, Rhazes, and Serapion,
Averroes, Damascenus, Constantine,
Bernard, and Gilbertus, and Gaddesden.
In his own diet he was temperate,
For it was nothing if not moderate,
Though most nutritious and digestible.
He didn't do much reading in the Bible.
He was dressed all in Persian blue and scarlet
Lined with taffeta and fine sarcenet,
And yet was very chary of expense.
He put by all he earned from pestilence:
In medicine gold is the best cordial.
So it was gold that he loved best of all.

Geoffrey Chaucer, *Canterbury Tales*,
trans. David Wright

Before the second doctor could be brought, the first
returned with the apothecary attending him as before.
He again surveyed and handled the sick; and when
Amelia begged him to tell her if there was any hope,
he shook his head, and said, 'To be sure, madam, miss is
in a very dangerous condition, and there is no time to
lose. If the blisters which I shall now order her, should
not relieve her, I fear we can do no more.' — 'Would
you not please, sir,' says the apothecary, 'to have the
powders and the draught repeated?' 'How often were
they ordered?' cries the doctor. 'Only *tertia quaq. hora*,'
says the apothecary. 'Let them be taken every hour by
all means,' cries the doctor; 'and — let me see, pray
get me a pen and ink.' — 'If you think the child in

such imminent danger,' said Booth, 'would you give us leave to call in another physician to your assistance — indeed my wife' — 'Oh, by all means,' said the doctor, 'it is what I very much wish. Let me see, Mr Arsenic, whom shall we call?' 'What do you think of Dr Dosewell?' said the apothecary. — 'Nobody better,' cries the physician. — 'I should have no objection to the gentleman,' answered Booth, 'but another hath been recommended to my wife.' He then mentioned the physician for whom they had just before sent. 'Who, sir?' cries the doctor, dropping his pen; and when Booth repeated the name of Thompson, 'Excuse me, sir,' cries the doctor hastily, 'I shall not meet him.' — 'Why so, sir?' answered Booth. 'I will not meet him,' replied the doctor. 'Shall I meet a man who pretends to know more than the whole College, and would overturn the whole method of practice, which is so well established, and from which no one person hath pretended to deviate?' 'Indeed, sir,' cries the apothecary, 'you do not know what you are about, asking your pardon; why, he kills everybody he comes near.' 'That is not true,' said Mrs Ellison. 'I have been his patient twice, and I am alive yet.' 'You have had good luck, then, madam,' answered the apothecary, 'for he kills everybody he comes near.' 'Nay, I know above a dozen others of my own acquaintance,' replied Mrs Ellison, 'who have all been cured by him.' 'That may be, madam,' cries Arsenic; 'but he kills everybody for all that — why, madam, did you never hear of Mr —? I can't think of the gentleman's name, though he was a man of great fashion; but everybody knows whom I mean.' 'Everybody, indeed, must know whom you mean,' answered Mrs Ellison; 'for I never heard but of one, and that many years ago.'

Before the dispute was ended, the doctor himself entered the room. As he was a very well-bred and very good-natured man, he addressed himself with much civility to his brother physician, who was not quite so courteous on his side. However, he suffered the newcomer to be conducted to the sick-bed, and at Booth's earnest request to deliver his opinion.

The dispute which ensued between the two physicians would, perhaps, be unintelligible to any but those of the faculty, and not very entertaining to them. The character which the officer and Mrs Ellison had given of the second doctor had greatly prepossessed Booth in his favour, and indeed his reasoning seemed to be the juster. Booth therefore declared that he would abide by his advice, upon which the former operator, with his zany, the apothecary, quitted the field, and left the other in full possession of the sick.

The first thing the new doctor did was (to use his own phrase) to blow up the physical magazine. All the powders and potions instantly disappeared at his command; for he said there was a much readier and nearer way to convey such stuff to the vault, than by first sending it through the human body. He then ordered

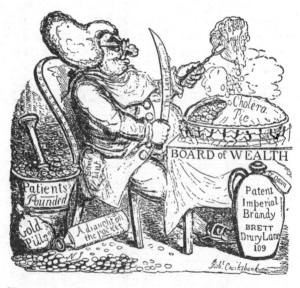

Nineteenth-century caricature illustrating a popular belief that physicians grew rich from epidemics.

the child to be blooded, gave it a clyster and some cooling physic, and, in short (that I may not dwell too long on so unpleasing a part of history) within three days cured the little patient of her distemper, to the great satisfaction of Mrs Ellison, and to the vast joy of Amelia.

Henry Fielding, *Amelia*, 1751

The 'good' doctor has certainly not invariably benefited financially, as this anecdote concerning the eighteenth-century London quack, Rock, amusingly demonstrates.

He was standing one day at his door on Ludgate Hill when a real Doctor of Physic passed, a man who had learning and abilities but whose modesty was the true cause of his poverty. 'How comes it,' says he to the Quack, 'that you without education, without skill, without the least knowledge of science, are enabled to live in the style you do? — You keep your town house, your carriage and your country house: whilst I, allowed to possess some knowledge, have neither, and can hardly pick up a subsistence!' 'Why look ye,' said Rock smiling, 'how many people do you think have passed since you asked me that question?' 'Why,' answered the Doctor, 'perhaps a hundred.' 'And how many of those hundred, think you, possess common sense?' 'Possibly one,' answered the Doctor. 'Then,' said Rock, 'that one comes to you; and I take care of the other ninety-nine.'

Quoted in James George Semple, *Memoirs*, 1787

Sometimes, of course, the Quack and the Doctor are one and the same person. Such was the eighteenth-century 'healer', Dr James Graham, who opened a Medical Institute (The Temple of Health) in 1780 in Pall Mall. It contained a magneto-electric bed where those suffering from infertility could 'infallibly produce a genial and happy issue'. Graham maintained that his bed could not only cure the barren but those procreating on it would enjoy orgasms prolonged to hours.

Here is a contemporary account by a French visitor to Dr Graham's Medical Institute.

Scarcely has one set foot on the first step on the staircase than one hears harmonious strains of wind instruments which reach the ear through hidden openings in the staircase, while the sweetest perfumes flatter the sense of smell till the entrance of a magnificent apartment is reached. This is used for the delivery of lectures in which the Doctor professes to abolish barrenness. Music precedes each lecture from five o'clock till seven when Dr Graham presents himself vested in doctor's robes. On the instant, there follows a silence which is interrupted only at the end of the lecture by an electric shock given to the whole audience by means of conductors hidden under the cushions with which all the seats are covered. . . All these details, however, are only accessories of his establishment. The sumptuous bed in brocaded damasks is supported by four crystal pillars of spiral shape. On whatever side one gets into this bed, which is called Celestial, one hears an organ played in unison with three others which make agreeable

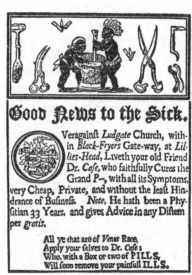

Good News to the Sick.

Veragainſt *Ludgate* Church, within *Black-Fryers* Gate-way, at *Lillies-Head*, Liveth your old Friend Dr. *Caſe*, who faithfully Cures the Grand P—, with all its Symptoms, very Cheap, Private, and without the leaſt Hindrance of Buſineſs. *Note*, He hath been a Phyſitian 33 Years, and gives Advice in any Diſtemper *gratis*.

All ye that are of *Venus* Race,
Apply your ſelves to Dr. *Caſe* :
Who, with a Box or two of PILLS,
Will ſoon remove your painfull ILLS.

music consisting of varied airs which carry the happy couples into the arms of Morpheus. For nearly an hour that the concert lasts one sees, in the bed, streams of light which play especially over the pillars. When the time for getting up has come, the magician comes to feel the pulse of the faithful, gives them breakfast, and sends them away full of hope, not forgetting to recommend them to send him other clients.

Quoted in Eric Jameson, *The Natural History of Quacks*

The 'quack' doctor is justly associated with metropolitan life and fashion. The country doctor has a much better press — called out as he is only when strictly necessary.

Anyone who has lived in these mountain regions knows what sickness means there. There are miles of track, broken and rutted by the winter rains, before you even reach the high road. The people there never send for medical aid for petty ailments. The doctor is not even summoned for important family events. He is only called in when life is in jeopardy. Here in this district you have fifty square miles without a doctor. Ask anybody who has lived on a wayside farm in these districts or in the villages in the valleys and they will tell you that one of the most vivid memories of their youth was to be wakened up in the dead of night by hearing the clatter of a horse ridden furiously past in the dark, and everyone knew there was a dire struggle for life going on in the hills.

David Lloyd George, House of Commons speech, 1912

The country doctor who is called out may not be master of the situation as others may assume. He could be young and inexperienced.

My patient continued to get worse and worse. You, my good sir, are not a doctor; you have no idea of what goes on inside a doctor's head, especially in his early days, when it dawns on him that a patient's illness is defeating him. All his self-assurance vanishes into thin air. I can't tell you how scared he gets. It seems to him that he's forgotten everything he ever knew, that his patient has no confidence in him, that other people are beginning to notice that he's out of his depth, and don't want to describe the patient's symptoms, that they are looking at him strangely, and whispering . . . oh, it's terrible. He feels there must be some way of treating the case if only it could be found. Perhaps this is it? He tries — no, wrong after all. He leaves no time for the treatment to take its proper effect . . . he snatches first at one method, then at another. He takes up his book of prescriptions . . . here it is, he thinks, this is it! To be quite honest sometimes he opens the book at random: this, he thinks, must be the hand of fate. . . Meanwhile there is someone dying; someone whom another doctor might have saved. I must have another opinion, you think; I won't take the whole responsibility myself. But what a fool you look on such occasions! Well, as time goes on, you get used to it, you say to yourself: never mind. The patient has died — it's not your fault; you only followed the rules. But what disturbs you still more is this: when other people have blind confidence in yourself, and all the time you know that you're helpless.

Ivan Turgenev, *A Sportsman's Sketches*, 1847–51

My favourite real nineteenth-century doctor was one much nearer home — my home — one Dr William Price, who was a great eccentric. Sometimes he walked about naked or else was fantastically garbed in a green and blue costume, performing Druidic rites. But he was a skilful doctor and surgeon, a socialist and free-thinker, one who early advocated cremation. When he was eighty-one he called his new-born son, Jesus Christ. Alas, the child died. . .

No one was prepared for the dreadful act he now per-petrated in a walled field he owned above the village at the very time when the Llantrisant chapel was con-ducting a Christian service below. The act roused to full fury the latent hostility he had earned in the past from most of the locality. It was also to bring him wide fame, in addition to posthumous canonization by the Cremation Society of Great Britain. The date was 13 January 1884. The father carried his son's body, wrapped in linen, to the field called Caerlan. A cask of paraffin waited there. Dr Price lit a wide ring of fire about this altar, placed the body on the cask, and set a torch to the oil. He remained chanting within the circle of fire. But news of his blasphemous intention had quickly spread and men were assembling; by the time the chapel had emptied others were speeding up to the field, some armed with sticks and cudgels. The police had also been informed. Two constables hurried up, arriving in time to prevent the unmoved doctor from being assaulted, if not lynched; they drew their batons. One constable, cape over head, dashed to the cask and snatched out the half-burned body.

Dr Price was taken into custody and conveyed to Pontypridd police station — for his own safety, the police later contended. The whole district was set by the ears. But the doctor, released after one night's detention, remained unruffled. At an inquest on the body the coroner found himself unable to grant permission to the police to bury it. Dr Price was claiming ownership, and also refusing not to attempt cremation again — 'I am not asking you to return to me the body of my child,' he said. 'I am demanding it.' The body was returned to him. Ignoring the dangerous hostility he had roused and denounced from pulpits all over Wales, he carried the cremation through some weeks later at the same spot. He was not molested. It was known that a legal prosecution of him was being instituted. But that night a mob attacked his cottage with stones. Shouting figures called on the old heretic to come out and face them. Suddenly the door opened and Gwenllian Llewyllyn [his wife] appeared, a pistol in each hand. She threatened to shoot. The mob dispersed.

Price was indicted at the next Cardiff assizes, for cremating the dead body of a child. Dressed in a snowy linen robe and a coloured shawl, he spoke in court with his usual eloquence and legal knowledge. The case became famous throughout the world. Mr Justice Stephen ruled that cremation of the dead was not illegal provided that it was carried out in such a manner as not to constitute a public nuisance at common law. After his acquittal, Price instituted proceedings against the Pontypridd police for false imprisonment and was awarded damages. He also caused a commemoration medal of the cremation to be struck, and sold thousands of these at threepence each.

Rhys Davies, *Print of a Hare's Foot*, 1969

Medicine practised in nineteenth-century Britain may have been, by our lights, somewhat primitive, but what of the present-day healers in the Third World? Many may well be like Raimi Agbonijo who practises traditional medicine in Ibadan.

Raimi Agbonijo is an older man, in his mid-sixties, and he announces himself as an established herbalist of some repute. His fame, he declares, is widespread and he has been as far afield as Ghana, Dahomey and the Cameroons, where his services are much in demand.

As a precaution in an encounter with someone who professes another brand of medicine, Mr Agbonijo wears a talismanic brass ring specially prepared for the occasion and he also has his curing apparatus handy. This magical instrument consists of unspecified materials tightly rolled into a ball of black cloth tied about with white thread. Had the occasion demanded it, he would have 'blown' a powerful curse across it in the direction of the author. . .

His education began when he was eight years of age, and he still continues it. Now he himself has taken on apprentices, but any serious healer should continue to acquire knowledge from other specialists. 'However strong the healer he cannot cure himself,' he warns and in the event of his own sickness he would be obliged to seek help elsewhere, possibly from a series of other doctors.

Whilst he believes that any good herbalist should be able to divine, he personally does not employ any systematic method, claiming instead a facility for direct diagnosis. He would regard it as absurd to discuss the nature of an illness with a patient; as the doctor, he can discern both cause and cure, whereas the patient knows nothing.

Apparently if someone approaches for a consultation he first makes a rapid assessment to decide whether he can cure the condition. Then he confronts the patient with the cost and usually demands payment in advance.

He mentions the treatment of *warapa* (major epileptic fits in an adult). This he explains is a disease brought about by the evil intentions of an enemy who has placed a medicine on the victim's clothing. Provided that the substance has come into contact with a garment, whether or not it is being worn at the time, epilepsy will ensue and will persist until the appropriate very costly therapeutic process has caused the patient to vomit up a live lizard.

A still more serious condition is *ete* (leprosy), which Mr Agbonijo also claims to treat. He emphasizes that the patient must meanwhile live in isolation in the bush to avoid contagion and he has a number of ideas about its causation, feeling that it may be hereditary, or perhaps spread through a family by spiders but, in an individual case, it may be a punishment for adultery.

His opinions about tuberculosis are a blend of traditional and modern. He quotes the common Ibadan belief that it is the disease spread by a chewing stick, adding the refinement that he thinks it is due to a fly landing on the stick. But he also states that it is spread by coughing and exacerbated by drinking local gin.

Dr Una Maclean, *Magical Medicine*, 1971

Western-trained doctors in the Third World countries
are not always the most efficient. Some are more
dangerous than the local witch-doctors. Too many are
like the Bulgarian, Dr Kostov, who practised obstetrics
in Algeria. Ian Young, a medical student, spent a
summer working alongside him in an Algerian pro-
vincial maternity unit.

'In Bulgaria,' says Dr Kostov, 'doctors never wait.'
I'm back in the world I was in before Calie arrived, sitting next to Dr Kostov on a Theatre stool. Neither of
us wears a mask, neither of us wears overshoes. The
hospital hasn't any. We're waiting for the instrument
orderly to arrive. The girl on the table has nice veins.
A second orderly is putting up a drip. He's the anaesthetist. The bottle contains normal saline, and comes
from France. The giving-set is West German, and the
needle's from Poland. With some tape and ingenuity, it
can all be fitted together. The orderly's had plenty of
practice. He'll be keeping the girl asleep with intravenous barbiturates. The hospital ran out of anaesthetic
gas a month ago.

I ask Dr Kostov what the Caesarean is for. He tells
me the girl's being looked after by one of the private
doctors in town, the man with the diploma in obstetrics
and gynaecology. The doctor sent her into hospital this
afternoon because she'd started bleeding. In his note,
he said she was eight months pregnant. He suspected
a placenta previa. That means, says Dr Kostov, that
instead of being at the back of her womb, the girl's
placenta has taken root over her cervix. For the baby
to be born, it would have to push its way through its
own placenta. That's why she needs a Caesarean. I ask
him if he could actually feel the placenta through the
cervix. Probably, he says, but it was Djamila who
examined the girl.

On the girl's chart under the heading 'Examination',
there's an empty space. The chart only gives her name
and her age, eighteen. She's brown and slim and naked.

For eight months, her belly's small. Her arms are strapped to a crosspiece that runs under her shoulders, and her thighs are held with clamps. She has a necklace, and bracelets round each wrist, from the jewellers of Beni Yenni in the mountains. Red and blue coral, set in silver. The soles of her feet are a deep orange, stained with henna. Her black hair has been brought back in two tight plaits, wound with green cloth. The Theatre light shines down on her belly, where the incision's to be made, and she groans a little as she breathes. 'Lebess?' cries Dr Kostov from his stool. 'Lebess,' she whispers back.

The instrument orderly arrives, and I go next door with Dr Kostov to scrub up. Coats off, we're bare-chested. Brushes in antiseptic soap, feet on the pedals that work a tap of sterile water. We wash for several minutes in silence. We come back into Theatre with our hands up, pushing the door open with our feet, and put on the sterile gowns that have the face masks incorporated. The gloves are sterile too, but they're the old Polish autopsy kind, deformed by over-use, curling back at the wrists so there's an inch of skin between the end of your gown and the beginning of your glove.

We're expecting Djamila any minute. A table's ready for the baby laid with a cloth, next to the anaesthetic trolley. There's a rubber sucker for clearing fluid from its airway, and a little mask, in case oxygen's necessary. Djamila should also be bringing along the stethoscope, so that Dr Kostov can have a last listen to the baby's heart before going in. We're all gowned and ready to start. 'We won't wait for her,' decides Dr Kostov, 'on y va!' I ask him how the baby's heart sounded earlier. Probably good, he says, but it was Djamila who examined the girl.

He takes a swab and begins to clean the girl's belly with blue antiseptic. He suddenly realises she hasn't been shaved. Whose responsibility? Djamila's or ours now? It's a detail, decides Dr Kostov, and we lay sterile cloths over her body. The orderly injects a syringeful of thiopentone into the drip, and seconds later the girl's unconscious.

Dr Kostov goes in via a midline incision. It's jagged, but that's the scalpel's fault more than his. We leave the bleeding points, Caesareans have got to be quick. Out of the corner of my eye, I notice Djamila arrive, with a cloth for the baby. Dr Kostov's reached the womb. I have two clamps and a pair of scissors ready for the cord. He takes the scalpel again and makes a cut an inch or two long across the womb, in the ugly fashion that's proper to him and Dr Vasilev. Two strong forefingers pull the incision apart. His hand dives inside and I'm holding my two clamps open, ready. But there's no baby inside the womb. There's only a bunch of small red grapes — a collection of bloody caviar.

'Mole!' gasps Dr Kostov, lifting it out. 'Oh la la,' says Djamila, 'you won't be needing me any more.' The orderlies mutter after her as she leaves: 'A girl who chews gum.'

There's a strange tumour that carries the old-fashioned name of a 'mole'. The womb fills and the belly expands, as if there were a real baby inside. But a mole pregnancy is more difficult than a real one. The mother gets more tired and more sick. Her belly's larger than it should be. After only three months, a mole can look like an eight-month normal pregnancy. And instead of increasing constantly, its size will often vary from day to day. If you feel the womb you won't find a baby's head. If you listen to the belly, you won't hear a baby's heart. You don't treat a mole. It miscarries, usually around the third or fourth month, and the woman's soon back to normal. The one thing you never do is operate. You run the risk of spreading the tumour cells to the rest of the mother's body, allowing them to grow and multiply in her lungs and brain.

Dr Kostov pushes aside my fingers with a growl. I can't do anything right. I stay away, just swabbing blood here and there on the edge of the field. Dr

Kostov's beyond help from any quarter. The error he's made is so grotesque that even in his own eyes it must have expelled him from twentieth-century obstetrics. Instruments lie neglected on the tray beside him. He's forfeited the right to their use. He stares into his incision, as if paralysed.

Ian Young, *The Private Life of Islam*, 1974

Some of my most regrettable errors have been the result of not spending sufficient time to find out the real cause of the patient's suffering. A case in point. I once treated a patient for twenty years without finding out the real trouble. Not until her husband became my patient did the real facts become clear.

Arthur E. Hertzler, *The Horse and Buggy Doctor*

> Cur'd yesterday of my disease
> I died last night of my physician.
>
> Matthew Prior (1664–1721), 'The Remedy Worse
> than the Disease'

When my father was an intern, one of the attending physicians on the P & S medical service of Roosevelt Hospital was an elderly, highly successful pomposity of New York medicine, typical of the generation trained long before the influence of Sir William Osler. This physician enjoyed the reputation of a diagnostician, with a particular skill in diagnosing typhoid fever, then the commonest disease on the wards of New York's hospitals. He placed particular reliance on the appearance of the tongue, which was universal in the medicine of that day (now entirely inexplicable, long forgotten). He believed he could detect significant differences by palpating that organ. The ward rounds conducted by this man were, essentially, tongue rounds; each patient would stick out his tongue while the eminence took it between thumb and forefinger, feeling its texture and irregularities, then moving from bed to bed, diagnosing typhoid in its earliest stages over and over again, and turning out a week or so later to have been right, to everyone's amazement. He was a more productive carrier, using only his hands, than Typhoid Mary.

Lewis Thomas, *The Youngest Science*, 1984

Of all those who have mocked the profession of medicine, few have hit their targets more humorously than Swift and Molière.

I was going on to tell him of another sort of people, who get their livelihood by attending the sick; . . . and because I had some skill in the faculty, I would in gratitude to his Honour, let him know the whole mystery and method by which they proceed.

Their fundamental is, that all diseases arise from *Repletion*; from whence they conclude, that a great *Evacuation* of the *Body* is necessary, either through the natural passage, or upwards at the mouth. Their next business is from herbs, minerals, gums, oils, shells, salts, juices, sea-weed, excrements, barks of trees, serpents, toads, frogs, spiders, dead men's flesh and bones, birds, beasts and fishes, to form a composition for smell and taste the most abominable, nauseous and detestable, that they can possibly contrive, which the stomach immediately rejects with loathing: and this they call a *Vomit*. Or else from the same store-house, with some other poisonous additions, they command us to take in at the orifice *above* or *below* (just as the Physician then happens to be disposed) a medicine equally annoying and disgustful to the bowels; which relaxing the belly drives down all before it: and this they call a *Purge* or a *Clyster*. For Nature (as the Physicians allege) having intended the superior anterior orifice only for the *Intromission* of solids and liquids, and the inferior posterior for ejection; these artists ingeniously considering that in all diseases Nature is forced out of her seat; therefore to replace her in it, the body must be treated in a manner directly contrary, by interchanging the use of each orifice; forcing solids and liquids in at the anus, and making evacuations at the mouth.

Jonathan Swift, *Gulliver's Travels*, 1726

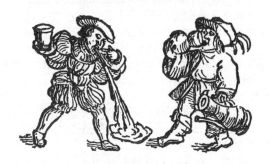

SGANARELLE. . . . In my opinion this impediment in the action of her tongue is caused by certain humours, which we savants call unhealthy humours, that is to say . . . unhealthy humours; seeing that the vapours formed by the exhalation of the influences which take rise in the seat of maladies, coming . . . so to speak . . . from . . . er. . . Do you understand Latin?

GÉRONTE. Not a word.

SGANARELLE [*rising abruptly*]. You don't know a word of Latin?

GÉRONTE. No.

SGANARELLE [*with enthusiasm*]. Cabricias arci thuram, catalamus, singulariter, nominativo, haec musa, the muse, bonus bona bonum. Deus sanctus, est-ne oratio latinas? Etiam, yes. Quare, why? Quia substantivo et adjectivum, concordat in generi, numerum et casus.

GÉRONTE. Oh, why didn't I study the arts?

JACQUELINE. There be a clever man for you!

LUCAS. Ay, by Gor, it be so fine I can't understand a word!

SGANARELLE. So these vapours, of which I am speaking, passing from the region of the liver on the left side to the region of the heart on the right, it happens that the lungs, which in Latin we call *armyan*, having communication with the brain, which in Greek we call *nasmus*, by means of the main artery, which in Hebrew we call *cubile*, meet on their way the said vapours which fill the ventricles of the shoulder-blade; and because the said vapours. . . Follow this closely if you please. . . And because the said vapours have a certain malign influence. . . Pay great attention to this, I beg of you.

GÉRONTE. Yes.

SGANARELLE. Have a certain malign influence, which is caused. . . Pay close attention, please.

GÉRONTE. I am.

SGANARELLE. Which is caused by the acridity of the humours engendered in the concavity of the diaphragm, it happens that these vapours . . . ossabandus, nequeis, nequer, potarinum, quipsa milus. There, that's the reason why your daughter is dumb.

JACQUELINE. Our doctor knows his business all right.

LUCAS. Would my tongue was as well oiled!

GÉRONTE. A clearer explanation would be impossible. There is only one thing which surprises me. That is the position of the liver and the heart. You seemed to me to place them the wrong way round. I always thought the heart was on the left side, and the liver on the right.

SGANARELLE. Yes, that used to be the case. But we have changed all that. The whole science of medicine is now run on an entirely new system.

> Molière, *Le Médecin malgré lui*, 1666,
> trans. George Graveley

A telling modern criticism, with its disturbing historical undertones, is implied in 'A Letter from Berlin' by Jon Stallworthy, whose father, a gynaecologist, might well have written a version of this letter just before the Second World War.

My dear,
      Today a letter from Berlin
where snow — the first of '38 — flew in,
settled and shrivelled on the lamp last night,
broke moth wings mobbing the window. Light
woke me early, but the trams were late:
I had to run from the Brandenburg Gate
skidding, groaning like a tram, and sodden
to the knees. Von Neumann operates at 10
and would do if the sky fell in. They lock
his theatre doors on the stroke of the clock —
but today I was lucky: found a gap
in the gallery next to a chap
I knew just as the doors were closing. Last,
as expected, on Von Showmann's list
the new vaginal hysterectomy
that brought me to Berlin.
               Delicately
he went to work, making from right to left
a semi-circular incision. Deft
dissection of the fascia. The blood-
blossoming arteries nipped in the bud.
Speculum, scissors, clamps — the uterus
cleanly delivered, the pouch of Douglas
stripped to the rectum, and the cavity
closed. Never have I seen such masterly
technique. 'And so little bleeding!' I said
half to myself, half to my neighbour.
               'Dead,'
came his whisper. 'Don't be a fool'
I said, for still below us in the pool
of light the marvellous unhurried hands
were stitching, tying the double strands
of catgut, stitching, tying. It was like
a concert, watching those hands unlock
the music from their score. And at the end
one half expected him to turn and bend
stiffly towards us. Stiffly he walked out
and his audience shuffled after. But

finishing my notes in the gallery
I saw them uncover the patient: she
was dead.

  I met my neighbour in the street
waiting for the same tram, stamping his feet
on the pavement's broken snow, and said:
'I have to apologize. She was dead,
but how did you know?' Back came his voice
like a bullet ' — saw it last month, twice.'

Returning your letter to an envelope
yellower by years than when you sealed it up,
darkly the omens emerge. A ritual wound
yellow at the lip yawns in my hand;
a turbulent crater; a trench filled
not with snow only, east of Buchenwald.

Jon Stallworthy, Root and Branch, 1969

Of course most doctors are caring — not cynical and
not ignorant. That is why most patients are grateful,
grateful to the doctors who treat them and the nurses
who nurse them.

Not that we all live up to the highest ideals, far from
it — we are only men. But we have ideals which mean
much, and they are realizable, which means more. Of
course there are Gehazis among us who serve for
shekels, whose ears hear only the lowing of the oxen
and the jingling of the guineas but these are exceptions;
the rank and file labour earnestly for your good, and
self-sacrificing devotion to your interest animates our
best work.

Sir William Osler, quoted in H. Cushing's Biography

It's the humdrum, day-in, day-out, everyday work
that is the real satisfaction of the practice of medicine;
the million and a half patients a man has seen on his
daily visits over a forty-year period of weekdays and
Sundays that make up his life. I have never had a
money practice; it would have been impossible for me.

But the actual calling on people, at all times and under all conditions, the coming to grips with the intimate conditions of their lives, when they were being born, when they were dying, watching them die, watching them get well when they were ill, has always absorbed me.

I lost myself in the very properties of their minds: for the moment at least I actually became *them*, whoever they should be, so that when I detached myself from them at the end of a half hour of intense concentration over some illness which was affecting them, it was as though I were reawakening from a sleep. For the moment I myself did not exist, nothing of myself affected me. As a consequence I came back to myself, as from any other sleep, rested.

William Carlos Williams, *Autobiography*, 1948

Today, at the medical school and hospital at which I teach and see patients, a brand-new intern told me the following story. While climbing a flight of stairs after the first full day of his internship, he met on the landing, coming down, an elderly man, bent and with a cane, but with the predictable shiningly alert eyes. The old man asked, 'Are you an intern?' On hearing the young doctor's tired, 'Yes,' the old man followed up with another question: 'Do you know what it takes to be a good intern?' 'No sir, I don't.' 'Well, it takes the heart of a lion, the eye of an eagle, and the hand of a lady.'

John Stone in *My Medical School*, 1978

Good Patients, Better Patients

1ST STUDENT. He's a bad patient, sir.

SIR ADOLPH ABRAHAMS. No such thing, boy, as a bad patient.

2ND STUDENT. Dr Lloyd said there were two kinds of patients.

SIR ADOLPH. What are they, boy?

2ND STUDENT. Rich patients and poor patients, sir.

Heard on a ward round, Westminster Hospital, 1946

We wait our turn, as still as mice,
For medicine free, and free advice:
Two mothers, and their little girls
So small — each one with flaxen curls —
And I myself, the last to come.
Now as I entered that bare room,
I was not seen or heard; for both
The mothers — one in finest cloth,
With velvet blouse and crocheted lace,
Lips painted red, and powdered face;
The oher ragged, whose face took
Its own dull, white, and wormy look —
Exchanged a hard and bitter stare.
And both the children, sitting there,
Taking example from that sight,
Made ugly faces, full of spite.
This woman said, though not a word
From her red painted lips was heard —
'Why have I come to this, to be
In such a slattern's company?'
The ragged woman's look replied —
'If you can dress with so much pride,
Why are you here, so neat, and nice,
For medicine free, and free advice?'

[44]

And I, who needed richer food,
Not medicine, to help my blood;
Who could have swallowed then a horse,
And chased its rider round the course,
Sat looking on, ashamed, perplexed,
Until a welcome voice cried — 'Next!'

W. H. Davies, 1928

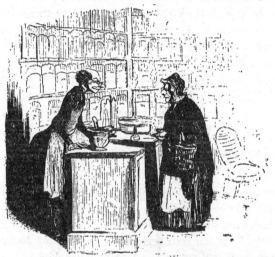

Sometimes the personal tragedy of a patient is overwhelming. For instance, a young mother brought her child into the Casualty Department to be circumcised. An anaesthetic was administered — fortunately not by myself. The child never woke up.

The mother waited on a bench outside the Casualty operating theatre, reading a magazine. The child lay dead on the table inside, and nothing would revive it. It won't take a few minutes, the nurse had told the mother. Breathe in, breathe out, there's a feller, the doctor had said to the child. The child breathed in and breathed out, then stopped breathing forever. It was an act of God. They had to tell her the child was dead. No, doctor, you don't understand, my husband doesn't know I brought our son to be circumcised. I did it without his permission. My husband was against the boy being circumcised. They stood there in white coats trying to explain to her again that the boy was dead. She would have to go home without her child — tell her husband, who did not know she had brought the child to the hospital in the first place. The mother had signed a form giving her permission for her child to be anaesthetised. The child proved to be allergic to the anaesthetic. A rare occurrence. So sorry. We're so very sorry. So rare for a patient to react to an anaesthetic like that. The mother comes into Casualty smiling, the child alive. The mother leaves without the child. The mother is crying. Next patient, please.

Dannie Abse, *A Poet in the Family*, 1974

Most patients have happier experiences even when their doctor makes a mistake — as in Mary Remmel's case.

9 June 1982

In three months time I shall be forty-nine years of age; last week I gave birth to a baby girl, our third child, a fact which I was informed of on 11 March.

No, I had not been negligent. I had seen my doctor way back in October last year and told him that I thought I could be pregnant. His response was to smile gently, tell me that if I was, I should make the headlines in our local paper. At my age pregnancy was just not possible, he said.

No test was made and I went away from the surgery somewhat relieved. After all he was a doctor; he had seen many women of my age in his career and I reasoned that he should know what the chances were.

Then I began to put on weight. My hands and ankles became swollen and I avidly read books on the change of life. There was nothing in them exactly like my symptoms but some of the things they said were near enough so I tried to rationalize the situation. I began next to worry that I might have a growth of some description. If I died of cancer what would my family do?

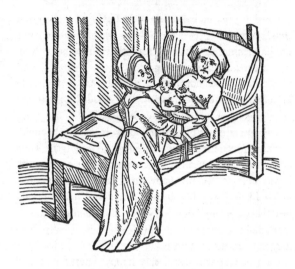

At last, when I could no longer fit any of my clothes and could hardly walk at anything but a crawl I went back to the surgery. This was in February. My doctor again said that it was nothing but my age, that I should go on a diet and that he would give me tablets for water retention.

I took the tablets, stuck to my diet and lost weight — that is, most of me lost weight. My tummy didn't, and I became more and more certain that I was carrying a child. I decided that if I were pregnant, I would seek an abortion. With my forty-ninth birthday coming up I thought this would be justified.

On 11 March therefore I went back to the surgery and saw another doctor, a woman. I told her of my fears. She examined me, the first examination I had had. Bluntly she informed me that I was seven months pregnant and that an abortion was out of the question.

I was glad I was lying down because I was shattered. She ushered me out of her room eventually with a prescription for iron tablets and the promise of an appointment with a specialist. I went automatically into town to do my shopping and as I did so felt differing emotions sweep through me. Anger that no one had listened to me, embarrassment at having to tell people that I was going to have a baby, shock that it could be happening at all and fear that in some way it might threaten our marriage.

Would it be normal? We both knew the risks attached to late pregnancies. We decided to tell our closest relatives and I shook each time.

The specialist confirmed the facts. It was, he thought, a viable pregnancy which could go to full term. I am apparently quite healthy and certainly not overweight. I was able to see my baby on a scan. It didn't look much like a baby but it was active and had a steady heartbeat. Seeing the baby on the monitor was a marvellous experience. I felt I knew it. I even held long conversations with it.

I am now serene and deeply happy where just a few weeks ago I was dominated by black despair. We have said goodbye to many of our old plans and are busy making new ones. We are also trying to adjust to the fact that we may often be mistaken for our child's grandparents in the not too distant future, but we have regained our sense of humour so I do not think this will bother us very much.

My life has a new purpose and I never knew I had so many friends and well-wishers. My marriage is more wonderful than ever and my husband and I are closer than we have ever been.

I realize how very lucky I am. Not every woman who finds herself in the same position at the same age is as fortunate, so I hope that any doctor who reads this will at least listen and find out that her fears are either groundless, or at least grounds for her to make a decision about how the rest of her life shall be ordered.

Mary Remmel, *The Times*

Mary Remmel's doctor had made the mistake partly because one patient in every three coming to his surgery suffered from a functional or stress disorder.

Nevertheless, non-organic symptoms may be very distressing, even alarming.

'This invisible wound hurts me terribly and I want you to cut out just that round part as far as the bone.'

'I am not going to do it, sir.'

'Why not?'

'Because there is nothing the matter with your hand. It is as healthy as my own.'

'You seem to think I am a madman, or that I am deceiving you,' said the patient as he drew out of his wallet a thousand-florin banknote and placed it on the table. 'You see I am in earnest. The matter is important enough for me to pay a thousand for it. Please perform the operation.'

'If you offered me all the money in the world I would not touch a healthy limb with the operating knife.'

'Why not?'

'Because it would not be according to professional ethics. All the world would call you an idiot and would accuse me of taking advantage of your weakness, or declare that I could not diagnose a wound that did not exist.'

'Very well, sir. Then I shall ask you another favour. I shall undertake the operation myself, though my left hand is rather clumsy at such things. All I will ask of you is to take care of the wound after I operate on it.'

The surgeon saw with astonishment that the man was quite serious and watched him take off his coat and turn up his shirt-sleeve. The man even took out his pocket knife, for want of any other instrument. Before the doctor could intervene, the stranger had made a deep incision in his hand.

'Stop,' he shouted, afraid lest the sufferer should sever a vein. 'Since you believe it must be done, very well, I'll do it.'

He then prepared for the operation. When it came to the actual cutting the doctor advised his patient to turn his head away, for people are generally upset at the sight of their own blood.

'Quite unnecessary,' said the other. 'I must direct your hand so that you may know how far to cut.'

The stranger took the operation stoically and was helpful with his directions. His hand never even trembled, and when the round spot had been carved out he sighed a happy sigh of relief, as if a load had been taken off his shoulders.

'You don't feel any pain now?' asked the surgeon.

'Not the least,' he said with a smile. 'It is as if the pain had been cut off and the slight irritation caused by the cutting seems like a cool breeze after a hot spell. Just let the blood run. It soothes me.'

After the wound was bandaged, the stranger looked happy and contented. He was a changed man. He gratefully pressed the doctor's hand with his own left hand.

'I am very grateful to you, indeed.'

The surgeon visited the patient at his hotel for several days after the operation and learned to respect the man, who occupied a high position in the county. He was learned and cultured, and was a member of one of the best families in the land.

After the wound was completely healed the stranger returned to his country home.

Three weeks later the patient again appeared in the surgeon's office. His hand was again in a sling and he complained of the same tormenting pain in the very spot where it hurt him before the operation.

Karoly Kisfaludi (1788–1830), *The Invisible Wound*
from *Great Short Stories of the World*, 1926

5 October 1897. To wake up at midnight after an hour's sleep, with a headache, slight but certainly indicative of the coming attack; to hear the clock strike, every note drilling a separate hole into your skull; to spend the rest of the night uneasily between sleeping and waking, always turning over the pillow, and tormented intermittently by idiotic nightmares, crowded with action which fatigues the brain; this is a distressed liver. Towards morning comes the hope, caused by the irregularity of the pain, that the headache will pass away on getting up. But it never does.

15 February 1911. I suspect that I have been working too hard for five weeks regularly. I feel an uncomfortable physical sensation all over the top of my head. A very quick sweating walk of half an hour will clear it off, but this may lead, and does lead, to the neuralgia of fatigue, and insomnia and so on, and I have to build myself up again with foods.

Arnold Bennett, *Journals*, 1932

I am reminded of the hypochondriac in a Clive Sinclair short story who seems to be suffering from 'introspective paranoia', of Molière's Monsieur Argan, and of the valetudinarian letter received, if not composed, by Joseph Addison in 1711.

It is six in the morning. Through my window I can see that the Vltava is turning gold with the rising of the sun. A beautiful sight, but I am immune to it; it fails to excite a single response in me. All it means is that it is time to move my bowels and to dress. Some days I am constipated, other days I have diarrhoea, less often I am regular. Every morning I examine the lavatory bowl, like an ancient sage, to see if I can divine what sort of a day I have in store. This is fundamentally much more important than either the weather or the view. Today my movements have been very loose, which means I must pass the hours between now and bedtime in constant anticipation of further activity, presaging who knows what stomach complaint.

Once I discussed this morbid hypochondria with a doctor acquaintance and he, priding himself on his psychological insight, said that I did not trust my own body, would not believe that all those millions of interdependent functions could go on performing in harmony day after day without supervision. He accused me of introspective paranoia.

Clive Sinclair, Hearts of Gold, 1979

ARGAN. Don't show your ignorance, girl. My apothecary's the best in Paris; and my doctor a man of the greatest skill, and learning — what he doesn't know about illnesses. . .

TOINETTE. I agree with you there. He smells 'em out, where nobody else would think of 'em.

ARGAN [*pleased*]. That's true; that's very true.

TOINETTE. Why, if it wasn't for him you wouldn't know you were ill.

ARGAN. That's true, that's . . . What are you talking about? Of course I should be ill, but I shouldn't know what *of*. When I wanted to talk of my illnesses I shouldn't know what to call 'em.

TOINETTE. Oh, your illnesses! They're all your little darlings, aren't they? With their own pet names — [*she waves an arm at the row of bottles*] — and each with a little bottle of its own — and when they're thirsty you give 'em drinks.

ARGAN. May you be forgiven! With all I have to suffer, I think this lack of sympathy is the hardest to bear.

Molière, Le Malade imaginaire, 1673, adaptation
by Miles Malleson, 1959

SIR,

I am one of that sickly tribe who are commonly known by the name of *Valetudinarians*, and do confess to you, that I first contracted this habit of body, or rather of mind, by the study of physick. I no sooner began to peruse books of this nature, but I found my pulse was irregular, and scarce ever read the account of any disease that I did not fancy myself afflicted with. Dr Sydenham's learned treatise of fevers threw me into a lingering hectic, which hung upon me all the while I was reading that excellent piece. I then applied myself to the study of several authors, who have written upon phthisical distempers, and by that means fell into à

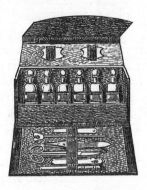

consumption, 'till at length, growing very fat, I was in a manner shamed out of that imagination. Not long after this I found in myself all the symptoms of the gout, except pain, but was cured of it by a treatise upon the gravel, written by a very ingenious author, who (as it is usual for physicians to convert one distemper into another) eased me of the gout by giving me the stone. I at length studied myself into a complication of distempers; but accidentally taking into my hand that ingenious discourse written by Sanctorius, I was resolved to direct myself by a scheme of rules, which I had collected from his observations. The learned world are very well acquainted with that gentleman's invention; who, for the better carrying on of his experiments, contrived a certain mathematical chair, which was so artificially hung upon springs, that it would weigh anything as well as a pair of scales. By this means he discovered how many ounces of his food passed by perspiration, what quantity of it was turned into nourishment, and how much went away by the other channels and distributions of nature. . .

I allow myself, one night with another, a quarter of a pound of sleep within a few grains more or less; and if upon my rising I find that I have not consumed my whole quantity, I take out the rest in my chair. Upon an exact calculation of what I expended and received last year, which I always register in a book, I find the medium to be two hundredweight, so that I cannot discover that I am impaired one ounce in my health during a whole twelvemonth. And yet, Sir, notwithstanding this my great care to ballast myself equally every day, and to keep my body in its proper poise, so it is that I find myself in a sick and languishing condition. My complexion is grown very sallow, my pulse low, and my body hydropical. Let me therefore beg you, Sir, to consider me as your patient, and to give me more certain rules to walk by than those I have already observed, and you will very much oblige

Your Humble Servant.

Joseph Addison, 'Valetudinarians', *The Spectator*,
29 March 1711

We may smile hearing of such hypochondriacal symptoms. However we cannot but be moved when we hear the testimony of patients with real afflictions.

For six years past I have fallen into an incurable condition, aggravated by senseless physicians, year after year deceived in the hope of recovery, and in the end compelled to contemplate a *lasting malady*, the cure of which may take years or even prove impossible. Born with a fiery lively temperament, inclined even for the amusements of society, I was early forced to isolate myself to lead a solitary life. If now and again I tried for once to give the go-by to all this, O how rudely was I repulsed by the redoubled mournful experience of my defective hearing; but not yet could I bring myself to say to people 'Speak louder, shout, for I am deaf.' O how should I then bring myself to admit the weakness of *a sense* which ought to be more perfect in me than in others, a sense which I once possessed in the greatest perfection, a perfection such as few assuredly in my profession have yet possessed it in — O I cannot do it! forgive me then, if you see me shrink away when I would fain mingle among you. Double pain does my misfortune give me, in making me misunderstood. Recreation in human society, the more delicate passages of conversation, confidential outpourings, none of these are for me; all alone, almost only so much as the sheerest necessity demands can I bring myself to venture into society; I must live like an exile; if I venture into company a burning dread falls on me, the dreadful risk of letting my condition be perceived. So it was these last six months which I passed in the country, being ordered by my sensible physician to spare my hearing as much as possible. He fell in with what has now become almost my natural disposition, though sometimes, carried away by craving for society, I let myself be misled into it; but what humiliation when someone stood by me and heard a flute in the distance, and I heard *nothing*, or when someone heard *the herd-boy singing*, and again I heard nothing.

Ludwig von Beethoven quoted in A *Way with Words*, 1982

TO MRS THRALE

Bolt Court, Fleet Street, 19 June 1783

Dear Madam,

I am sitting down in no cheerful solitude to write a narrative which would once have affected you with tenderness and sorrow, but which you will perhaps pass over now with the careless glance of frigid indifference. For this diminution of regard however, I know not whether I ought to blame you, who may have reasons which I cannot know, and I do not blame myself, who have for a great part of human life done you what good I could, and have never done you evil.

I had been disordered in the usual way, and had been relieved by the usual methods, by opium and cathartics, but had rather lessened my dose of opium.

On Monday the 16th I sat for my picture, and walked a considerable way with little inconvenience. In the afternoon and evening I felt myself light and easy, and began to plan schemes of life. Thus I went to bed, and in a short time waked and sat up, as has been long my custom when I felt a confusion and indistinctness in my head, which lasted I suppose about half a minute; I was alarmed, and prayed God, that however he might afflict my body, he would spare my understanding. This prayer, that I might try the integrity of my faculties I made in Latin verse. The lines were not very good, but I knew them not to be very good: I made them easily, and concluded myself to be unimpaired in my faculties.

Soon after I perceived that I had suffered a paralytic stroke, and that my speech was taken from me. I had no pain, and so little dejection in this dreadful state, that I wondered at my own apathy, and considered that perhaps death itself when it should come would excite less horror than seems now to attend it.

In order to rouse the vocal organs I took two drams. Wine has been celebrated for the production of eloquence. I put myself into violent motion, and I think repeated it; but all was vain. I then went to bed, and, strange as it may seem, I think, slept. When I saw light, it was time to contrive what I should do. Though God stopped my speech he left me my hand, I enjoyed a mercy which was not granted to my dear friend Lawrence, who now perhaps overlooks me as I am writing, and rejoices that I have what he wanted. My first note was necessarily to my servant, who came in talking, and could not immediately comprehend why he should read what I put into his hands.

I then wrote a card to Mr Allen, that I might have a discreet friend at hand to act as occasion should require. In penning this note I had some difficulty, my hand, I knew not how nor why, made wrong letters. I then wrote to Dr Taylor to come to me, and bring Dr Heberden, and I sent to Dr Brocklesby, who is my neighbour. My physicians are very friendly and very disinterested, and give me great hopes, but you may imagine my situation. I have so far recovered my vocal powers, as to repeat the Lord's Prayer with no very imperfect articulation. My memory, I hope, yet remains as it was; but such an attack produces solicitude for the safety of every faculty...

I suppose you may wish to know how my disease is treated by the physicians. They put a blister upon my back, and two from my ear to my throat, one on a side. The blister on the back has done little, and those on the throat have not risen. I bullied and bounced (it sticks to our last sand) and compelled the apothecary to make his salve according to the Edinburgh Dispensatory, that it might adhere better. I have two on now of my own prescription. They likewise give me salt of hartshorn, which I take with no great confidence, but am satisfied that what can be done is done for me.

O God! give me comfort and confidence in Thee; forgive my sins; and if it be Thy good pleasure, relieve my diseases for Jesus Christ's sake. Amen.

I am almost ashamed of this querulous letter, but now it is written, let it go.

I am, &c.,
Sam: Johnson

What is most remarkable is the courage of many patients — not only those who are stoical and considerate but those who conquer their fears through their own willed endeavours.

I was then in a state of health which furthered me sufficiently in all that I would and should undertake; only there was a certain irritability left behind, which did not always let me be in equilibrium. A loud sound was disagreeable to me, diseased objects awakened in me loathing and horror. But I was especially troubled with a giddiness which came over me every time I looked down from a height. All these infirmities I tried to remedy, and, indeed, as I wished to lose no time, in a somewhat violent way. In the evening when they beat the tattoo, I went near the multitude of drums, the powerful rolling and beating of which might have made one's heart burst in one's bosom. All alone I ascended the highest pinnacle of the minster spire, and sat in what is called the neck, under the nob or crown, for a quarter of an hour, before I would venture to step out again into the open air, where, standing upon a platform scarce an ell square, without any particular holding, one sees the boundless prospect before; while the nearest objects and ornaments conceal the church, and everything upon and above which one stands. It is exactly as if one saw one's self carried up into the air in a balloon. Such troublesome and painful sensations I repeated until the impression became quite indifferent to me; and I have since then derived great advantage from this training, in mountain travels and geological studies, and on great buildings, where I have vied with the carpenters in running over the bare beams and the cornices of the edifice, and even in Rome, where one must run similar risks to obtain a nearer view of important works of art. Anatomy, also, was of double value to me, as it taught me to endure the most repulsive sights, while I satisfied my thirst for knowledge. And thus I also attended the clinical course of the elder Doctor Ehrmann, as well as the lectures of his son on obstetrics, with the double view of becoming acquainted with all conditions, and of freeing myself from all apprehension as to repulsive things. And I have actually succeeded so far, that nothing of this kind could ever put me out of my self-possession.

Goethe, *Autobiography*, 1811–33,
trans. John Oxenford, 1848

The causes given in the following letter for Dylan Thomas's illnesses, are not in any textbook. It seems he failed to turn up to deliver a speech at the annual dinner of the British Medical Association's Swansea branch.

I plead that the collected will of the Members of the Swansea Branch of the British Medical Association, working by a clinically white magic known only to their profession, drove me, soon after my inexcusable non-appearance at their Annual Dinner, into a bag of sickness and a cropper of accidents from which I have not yet fully recovered. The first effect of this malevolent mass medical bedevilment I experienced a week after the dinner when stopping, heavily disguised, at Swansea in order to try to learn how really execrated I was in the surgeries and theatres, the bolus-rooms and Celtic lazarets of a town I can approach now only in the deepest dark and where certain areas, particularly around the hospital, are forever taboo to me. I felt sudden and excruciating pains, and when I whimpered about them to a friend he said, 'Whatever you do, don't get ill in Swansea, it's more than your life is worth. Go in with a cough and they'll circumcise you.' So I knew what the position was, and I took my pains home. But even at home, word of my unworthiness had reached the doctor's ears, and I was treated like a leper (fortunately, a wrong diagnosis). Ever since then I have felt unwell. A little later I had an attack of gout — undoubtedly the result of some Swansea specialist sticking a pin into a wax toe — and a little later still was set upon by invisible opponents in the bogled Laugharne dark and fell down and cracked my ribs.

Dylan Thomas, *Selected Letters*, 1966

Dylan Thomas was a Rabelaisian character. And when Rabelais' characters fall ill anything can happen.

A short time afterwards, our friend Pantagruel fell ill, being seized with such pains in his stomach that he was unable to eat or drink. And since troubles never come singly, he was afflicted at the same time with a burning of his urine, which caused him more agony than you might think. But his physicians took care of him, and very well, and made him piss away his pain with plenty of lenitive and diuretic drugs. His urine was so extremely hot that it has never cooled off, from that day to this. And as a result, you have in France today in various places where it ran, what are called hot-baths, as, for example:

At Cauterets;

At Limoux;

At Dax;

At Balaruc;

At Neris;

At Bourbon-Lancy and elsewhere.

In Italy:

At Monte Grotto;

At Abano;

At San Pietro of Padua;

At Sant' Elena;

At Casa Nuova;

At San Bartolomeo;

In the County of Bologna;

At Porretta, and a thousand other places.

And I am greatly astonished at a lot of foolish philosophers and physicians, who waste their time arguing about where the heat of these springs comes from, and whether it is due to borax, or to sulphur, or to alum, or to saltpetre in the ore, all they do is to concoct fairy stories, and it would be better for them to go scratch their arses on a thistle than to waste time in discussing something the origin of which they know nothing about. For the answer is easy, and there is no need of looking any further. The said baths are hot for the reason that they spring from the hot piss of our friend Pantagruel.

Rabelais (1494?–1553), *The Adventures of Gargantua and Pantagruel*, trans. Samuel Putnam

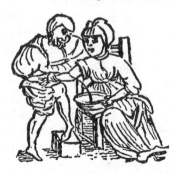

Rabelais was a doctor. And all doctors have some extra-
ordinary stories to tell about their patients. What about
this contemporary case-report from Dr J. O'Donnell, a
GP in Whitby, Yorkshire, who tells how one of his
patients sustained a Colles fracture of her left arm.

She and her husband had been attending a wedding reception, held in the house of a friend, and they had both
had too much to drink. The husband fell asleep on the
couch downstairs and a few minutes later his wife went
upstairs to a bedroom in order to sleep off the effects too.
The other guests were by now feeling very cheerful
and decided to have a bit of fun. They found the neck
of the turkey, the rest of which they had just eaten,
and placed it in the fly of the husband who was now
sound asleep on the couch.

The party broke up later on in the evening and the
other guests went home expecting to have a bit of a
giggle with the couple next day about the practical
joke they had played.

However the wife woke up at three o'clock in the
morning, not feeling very well, and went in search of
her husband. She went to the top of the stairs and saw
her husband lying on the couch with the cat on top
of him, gnawing cheerfully at the tasty morsel sticking
out of his fly. His wife leapt to the obvious conclusion,
fainted, fell downstairs, and fractured her arm.

J. O'Donnell, *World Medicine*, 14 November 1981

That fractured arm, of course, got better. The X-rays
soon showed the healing process had begun. Sometimes,
though, the X-ray report may be very serious indeed.
It can carry news that may be devastating.

DEVONSHIRE STREET W1

The heavy mahogany door with its wrought-iron screen
Shuts. And the sound is rich, sympathetic, discreet.
The sun still shines on this eighteenth-century scene
With Edwardian faience adornments — Devonshire
Street.

No hope. And the X-ray photographs under his arm
   Confirm the message. His wife stands timidly by.
The opposite brick-built house looks lofty and calm,
   Its chimneys steady against a mackerel sky.

No hope. And the iron nob of this palisade
   So cold to the touch, is luckier now than he.
'Oh merciless, hurrying Londoners! Why was I made
   For the long and the painful deathbed coming to
      me?'

She puts her fingers in his as, loving and silly,
   At long-past Kensington dances she used to do.
'It's cheaper to take the tube to Piccadilly
   And then we can catch a nineteen or a twenty-two.'

               John Betjeman, *Collected Poems*, 1980

Few patients, however, despite their condition, are devoid of hope. Almost all long for a miracle cure.

Some patients had achieved a state of icy hopelessness akin to serenity . . . they *knew* they were doomed, and they accepted this with all the courage and equanimity they could muster. Other patients (and, perhaps, to some extent, all of these patients, whatever their surface serenity) had a fierce and impotent sense of outrage: they had been *swindled* out of the best years of life; they were consumed by the sense of time lost, time *wasted*; and they yearned incessantly for a twofold miracle — not only a cure for their sickness, but an indemnification for the loss of their lives. They wanted to be given back the time they had lost, to be magically replaced in their youth and prime.

               Oliver W. Sacks, *Awakenings*, 1973

How he wanted to be cured! In spite of the numbing, obviously hopeless treatment, month after month and year after year — suddenly and finally to be cured! To have his back healed again, to straighten himself up, walk with a firm tread, be a fine figure of a man! 'Hallo, Ludmila Afanasyevna! I'm all right now!'

They all longed to find some miracle-doctor, or some medicine the doctors here didn't know about. Whether they admitted as much or denied it, they all without exception in the depths of their hearts believed there was a doctor, or a herbalist, or some old witch of a woman somewhere, whom you only had to find and get that medicine from to be saved.

No, it wasn't possible, it just wasn't possible that their lives were already doomed.

However much we laugh at miracles when we are strong, healthy and prosperous, if life becomes so hedged and cramped that only a miracle can save us, then we clutch at this unique, exceptional miracle and — believe in it!

Alexander Solzhenitsyn, Cancer Ward, 1968

But the last words about patients I would leave to the astute Charles Lamb.

If there be a regal solitude, it is a sick-bed. How the patient lords it there; what caprices he acts without control! how king-like he sways his pillow — tumbling, and tossing, and shifting, and lowering, and thumping, and flatting, and moulding it, to the ever-varying requisitions of his throbbing temples.

He changes *sides* oftener than a politician. Now he lies full length, then half length, obliquely, transversely, head and feet quite across the bed; and none accuses him of tergiversation. Within the four curtains he is absolute. They are his *mare clausum*.

How sickness enlarges the dimensions of a man's self to himself! he is his own exclusive object. Supreme selfishness is inculcated upon him as his only duty. 'Tis the Two Tables of the Law to him. He has nothing to think of but how to get well. What passes out of doors, or within them, so he hears not the jarring of them, affects him not. . .

To the world's business he is dead. He understands not what the callings and occupations of mortals are;

only he has a glimmering conceit of some such thing, when the doctor makes his daily call: and even in the lines on that busy face he reads no multiplicity of patients, but solely conceives of himself as *the sick man*. To what other uneasy couch the good man is hastening, when he slips out of his chamber, folding up his thin *douceur* so carefully, for fear of rustling — is no speculation he can at present entertain. He thinks only of the regular return of the same phenomenon at the same hour tomorrow.

Household rumours touch him not. Some faint murmur, indicative of life going on within the house, soothes him, while he knows not distinctly what it is. He is not to know anything, not to think of anything. Servants gliding up or down the distant staircase, treading as upon velvet, gently keep his ear awake, so long as he troubles not himself further than with some feeble guess at their errands. Exacter knowledge would be a burthen to him: he can just endure the presence of conjecture. He opens his eye faintly at the dull stroke of the muffled knocker, and closes it again without asking 'Who was it?' He is flattered by a general notion that enquiries are making after him, but he cares not to know the name of the enquirer. In the general stillness and awful hush of the house he lies in state, and feels his sovereignty.

To be sick is to enjoy monarchal prerogatives. Compare the silent tread and quiet ministry, almost by the eye only, with which he is served — with the careless demeanour, the unceremonious goings in and out (slapping of doors, or leaving them open) of the very same attendants, when he is getting a little better — and you will confess that from the bed of sickness (throne let me rather call it) to the elbow-chair of convalescence is a fall from dignity amounting to a deposition.

Charles Lamb, *The Convalescent*, from *Last Essays of Elia*, 1833

In Hospital

Something I should like to know is, which
    would everybody rather not do:
Be well and visit an unwell friend in the hospital,
    or be unwell in the hospital and have a well
    friend visit you?
This is a discussion which I am sorry that I ever
    commenced it,
For not only does it call up old unhappy memories,
    but each choice has so much to be said
    against it.
Take the sight of a visitor trying to entertain a
    patient or a patient trying to entertain a visitor,
It would bring joy to the heart of the Grand
    Inquisitor.
The patient is either too ailing to talk or is panting
    to get back to the chapter where the elderly
    spinster is just about to reveal to the Inspector
    that she now thinks she can identify the
    second voice in that doom-drenched quarrel.
And the visitor either has never had anything to
    say to the patient anyway or is wondering
    how soon it would be all right to depart for
    Belmont or Santa Anita or Laurel,
And besides, even if both parties have ordinarily
    much to discuss and are far from conversational
    mediocrities,
Why, the austere hygienic surroundings and the
    lack of ashtrays would stunt a dialogue between
    Madame de Staël and Socrates,
And besides, even if anybody did get to chatting
    glitteringly and gaudily,
They would soon be interrupted by the arrival
    of a nurse or an orderly.

It is a fact that I must chronicle with distress
That the repartee reaches its climax when the
    visitor finally spots the handle on the foot of
    the bed and cranks the patient's knees up and
    down and says, 'That certainly is ingenious,'
    and the patient answers Yes.
How many times a day do I finger my pulse and
    display my tongue to the mirror while waiting
    for a decision to be elicited:
Whether to ignore my host of disquieting
    symptoms and spend my days visiting friends
    who have surrendered to theirs, or to surrender
    to my own and spend my days being visited.

> Ogden Nash, 'Notes for the Chart in 306', from
> *There's Always Another Windmill*, 1968

A year ago I fell in love with the functional ward
Of a chest hospital: square cubicles in a row
Plain concrete, wash basins — an art lover's woe
Not counting how the fellow in the next bed snored.
But nothing whatever is by love debarred,
The common and banal her heat can know.
The corridor led to a stairway and below
Was the inexhaustible adventure of a gravelled
    yard.

This is what love does to things: the Rialto Bridge,
The main gate that was bent by a heavy lorry,
The seat at the back of a shed that was a suntrap.
Naming these things is the love-act and its pledge;
For we must record love's mystery without claptrap,
Snatch out of time the passionate transitory.

> Patrick Kavanagh, 'The Hospital', from *Collected Poems*,
> 1972

Whatever disadvantages a patient has to endure in a hospital nowadays — the fellow in the next bed snoring, etc. — is nothing to what our great-grandfather's grandfather's grandfather's grandfather had to put up with.

1650. 3 Of May, at the Hospital of the Charitie, I saw
the whole operation of Lithotomie namely 5 cut of the
stone: There was one person of 40 years old had a stone
taken out of him, bigger than a turkys Egg: The
manner thus: the sick creature was strip'd to his shirt,
and bound armes and thighs to an high Chaire, 2 men
holding his shoulders fast down: then the Chirurgion
with a crooked Instrument prob'd til he hit on the
stone, then without stirring the probe which had a
small channell in it, for the Edge of the Lancet to run
in, without wounding any other part, he made
Incision thro the Scrotum about an Inch in length,
then he put in his forefingers to get the stone as neere
the orifice of the wound as he could, then with another
Instrument like a Cranes neck he pull'd it out with
incredible torture to the Patient, especially at his after
raking so unmercifully up and downe the bladder with
a 3d instrument, to find any other Stones that may
possibly be left behind: The effusion of blood is greate.
Then was the patient carried to bed, and dress'd with
a silver pipe accommodated to the orifice for the urine
to passe, when the wound is sowed up: The danger is
feavor, and gangreene, some Wounds never closing:
and of this they can give shrewd conjecture by the
smothnesse or ruggednesse of the stone: The stone
pull'd forth is washed in a bason of water, and wiped
by an attendant Frier, then put into a paper and
writen on, which is also entred in a booke, with the
name of the person, shape, weight &c of the stone,
Day of the moneth, & Operator: After this person
came a little Child of not above 8 or 9 yeares age,
with much cherefullnesse, going through the operation
with extraordinary patience, and expressing greate joy,
when he saw the stone was drawn: The use I made of
it, was to give Almighty God hearty thankes, that I
had not ben subject to this Infirmitie, which is indede
deplorable.

The Diary of John Evelyn, ed. E. S. de Beer, 1959

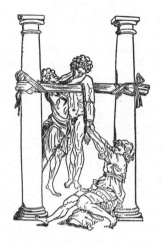

In the year 1709, when there were at least nine thousand people sleeping each night in the Hotel Dieu in Paris (the oldest hospital in Europe) there were only about one thousand beds there — six hundred large, and four hundred small — to accommodate them. Some of those beds may have contained as many as ten very sick invalids huddled uncomfortably together.

> Guy Williams, *The Age of Agony*, 1975

Some of the pre-Florence Nightingale nurses, too, were hardly tender. In London, in the oldest hospital in Britain, St Bartholomew's, during 1708, a Sister Owen and a Nurse Deane had to be reprimanded.

Sarah Owen Sister to Cathrines (St Catherine's) ward doth demand and take of every patient sent into that ward 2s 6d and causeth them to spend 6d: That Ann Deane her Helper likewise demands a Shilling of each patient and that the said Sister washeth her Sons and Daughters linnen and makes the patients Iron the same. Upon examining of Ann Preston, Martha Gold, Phillis Chamlett and Mary Browning now patients in that ward concerning the same Complaint they all declared that the said Sister and Helper do make such demands and that some patients have pawned their Cloths to raise money to satisfye them otherwise they are neglected and slighted. And that the same Sister doth cause her Sons and daughters linnen to be Iron'd by the patients.

Quoted in Guy Williams, *The Age of Agony*, 1975

It is a relief to hear of medical staff who are altogether more selfless — then and now.

I found the Children's Hospital established in an old sail-loft or store-house, of the roughest nature, and on the simplest means. There were trap-doors in the floors, where goods had been hoisted up and down; heavy feet and heavy weights had started every knot in the well-trodden planking; inconvenient bulks and beams and awkward staircases perplexed my passage through the wards. But I found it airy, sweet, and clean. In its seven-and-thirty beds I saw but little beauty; for starvation in the second or third generation takes a pinched look: but I saw the sufferings both of infancy and childhood tenderly assuaged; I heard the little patients answering to pet playful names; the light touch of a delicate lady laid bare the wasted sticks of arms for me to pity: the claw-like little hands, as she did so, twined themselves lovingly around her wedding-ring. . .

The nurses of this hospital are all young — ranging, say, from nineteen to four-and-twenty. They have even within these narrow limits what many well-endowed hospitals would not give them, a comfortable room of their own in which to take their meals. It is a beautiful truth, that interest in the children and sympathy with their sorrows, bind these young women to their places far more strongly than any other consideration could. The best skilled of the nurses came originally from a kindred neighbourhood, almost as poor; and she knew how much the work was needed. She is a fair dressmaker. The hospital cannot pay her as many pounds in the year as there are months in it; and one day the lady regarded it as a duty to speak to her about her improving her prospects, and following her

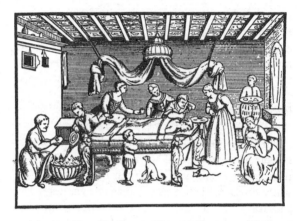

trade. No, she said: she could never be so useful or so happy elsewhere any more: she must stay among the children. And she stays. One of the nurses, as I passed her, was washing a baby boy. Liking her pleasant face, I stopped to speak to her charge — a common, bullet-headed, frowning charge enough, laying hold of his own nose with a slippery grasp, and staring very solemnly out of a blanket. The melting of the pleasant face into delighted smiles, as this young gentleman gave an unexpected kick, and laughed at me, was almost worth my previous pain.

An affecting play was acted in Paris years ago called 'The Children's Doctor'. As I parted from my children's Doctor now in question, I saw in his easy black necktie, in his loose buttoned black frock-coat, in his pensive face, in the flow of his dark hair, in his eyelashes, in the very turn of his moustache, the exact realisation of the Paris artist's ideal as it was presented on the stage. But no romancer that I know of has had the boldness to prefigure the life and home of this young husband and young wife in the Children's Hospital in the East of London.

I came away from Ratcliff by the Stepney railway station to the terminus at Fenchurch Street. Any one who will reverse that route may retrace my steps.

Charles Dickens, *The Uncommercial Traveller*, 1861

In the room a woman moves. She is dressed in white. Lovingly she measures his hourly flow of urine. With hands familiar, she delivers oxygen to his nostrils and counts his pulse as though she were telling beads. Each bit of his decline she records with her heart full of grief, shaking her head. At last, she turns from her machinery to the simple touch of the flesh. Sighing, she strips back the sheet, and bathes his limbs.

The man of letters did not know this woman before. Preoccupied with dying, he is scarcely aware of her presence now. But this nurse is his wife in his new life of dying. They are close, these two, intimate, depending one upon the other, loving. It is a marriage, for although they own no shared past, they possess this awful, intense present, this matrimonial now, that binds them as strongly as any promise.

A man does not know whose hands will stroke from him the last bubbles of his life. That alone should make him kinder to strangers.

Richard Selzer, *Mortal Lessons*, 1981

Not all modern nurses or, indeed, hospitals, are so caring. Some institutions in certain parts of the world remain backward, resembling the hospital in Chekhov's 'Ward Six', or the strange symbolic hospital depicted in Dino Buzzati's 'Seven Floors'.

When Andrei Yefimych came to our town to take up his duties, the 'charitable institution' was in an appalling state. One could hardly breathe for the stench in the wards, corridors and hospital yard. The hospital attendants, the nurses, and their children all slept in the wards with the patients. Everyone complained that life was made miserable by cockroaches, bedbugs and mice. In the surgical ward they had not yet got rid of erysipelas. There were only two scalpels in the entire hospital, not a single thermometer, and the bathtubs were used for storing potatoes. The superintendent, matron, and medical assistant all robbed the patients, and the old doctor, Andrei Yefimych's predecessor, was said to have engaged in the illicit sale of the hospital alcohol and to have organized a veritable harem for himself among the nurses and patients. The townspeople were well aware of these irregularities and even exaggerated them, but took them calmly; some justified them on the grounds that only peasants and workingmen went to the hospital, and they had nothing to complain of since they were considerably worse off at home – you wouldn't expect them to feed on woodcock! Others made the excuse that the town wasn't able to support a decent hospital without help from the zemstvo; thank God for any hospital, even a bad one! But the recently formed zemstvo failed to open a hospital either in the town or in the district on the grounds that the town already had one.

After inspecting the hospital, Andrei Yefimych came to the conclusion that it was an infamous institution, highly detrimental to the health of the community. In his opinion the wisest thing to do would be to discharge the patients and close the hospital. But for this, he reasoned, something more than his will would be required, and in any case it would serve no purpose; if physical and moral impurity were driven out of one place they would only move to another; one must wait for it to wither away of itself. Moreover, if the people had opened the hospital and tolerated it, it meant that they needed it: superstition and all the rest of life's filth and abominations are necessary, for in time they are converted into something useful, as dung into black soil. There is nothing on earth so fine that its origin is without foulness.

Once he had taken up his duties, Andrei Yefimych did not appear to be greatly concerned about the irregularities. He only asked the hospital attendants and nurses not to sleep in the wards and installed two cupboards of instruments; but the superintendent and the matron did not change, and the erysipelas in the surgical ward remained.

Anton Chekhov, *Ward Six*, trans. Ann Dunnigan, 1965

After the nurse left, Giuseppe Corte had an impression that his fever had gone; he went to the window, not so much to take in the view of the town, although it was new to him, as hoping to see other patients through the windows on the floor below. The structure of the building, with its spacious sunporches, allowed for such observation. Giuseppe Corte fixed his attention on the windows of the ground floor especially, which seemed very remote and could be seen only at an angle. But he saw nothing of interest. Most of them were shrouded in hermetic seclusion, behind silent venetian blinds.

Corte noticed that a man was leaning out of the window next to his. The two looked at each other for some time, with growing interest. But they found it hard to break the silence. At last Giuseppe Corte summoned his courage and said: 'Did you just arrive, too?'

'Oh no,' answered the other. 'I've been here two months already. . .' He was silent for a few minutes and not knowing how to continue the conversation, he added: 'I was looking for my brother down there.'

'Your brother?'

'Yes,' the unknown man explained, 'we arrived together. Really a very strange thing; he got worse and worse; think of it; he's on the fourth already.'

'On the fourth what?'

'On the fourth floor,' the man answered, and he pronounced the two words with an accent of such commiseration and horror that Giuseppe Corte remained as though transfixed.

'But is it so serious on the fourth floor?' he asked warily.

'O Lord,' said the other slowly, shaking his head. 'They're not hopeless yet, but it's nothing to be happy about.'

'But then,' Corte asked again with the joking casualness of one who touches on another man's tragedies, 'but in that case, if it's already so serious on the fourth floor, who do they put on the ground floor?'

'On the ground floor are the moribund. Down there nothing remains for the doctors. Only the priest works there. And of course. . .'

'But there aren't many on the ground floor,' Giuseppe Corte said suddenly as if eager for confirmation, 'nearly all the rooms there are closed.'

'There are only a few now, but this morning there were many more,' the stranger answered, with a subtle smile. 'Where the blinds are lowered, that's where someone has died. Don't you see that the windows are open on the other floors? But, excuse me,' he said, slowly withdrawing, 'it seems to be turning cold. I'm going back to bed. Good luck, good luck. . .'

The man stepped back from the window and closed it emphatically. Then a light went on inside. Giuseppe Corte remained stationary at the window, staring at the lowered blinds on the ground floor. He looked at them with queer intensity, trying to imagine the grim secrets of that fearful ground floor where the patients were kept to die; and he felt glad to know he was so far away from it. Meanwhile the evening shadows were falling. The thousand windows of the institution lit up, one by one; at a distance it might have been a palace ball. Only on the ground floor, at the bottom of the abyss, dozens and dozens of windows remained blind and dark.

Dino Buzzati, 'Seven Floors', from *Catastrophe and other stories*, 1965

Then there are mental hospitals which have their own particular atmosphere and imperatives.

The night attendant, a B.U. sophomore,
rouses from the mare's nest of his drowsy head
propped on *The Meaning of Meaning*.
He catwalks down our corridor.
Azure day
makes my agonized blue window bleaker.
Crows maunder on the petrified fairway.
Absence! My heart grows tense

as though a harpoon were sparring for the kill.
(This is the house for the 'mentally ill'.)

What use is my sense of humour?
I grin at 'Stanley', now sunk in his sixties,
once a Harvard all-American fullback
(if such were possible!),
still hoarding the build of a boy in his twenties,
as he soaks, a ramrod
with the muscle of a seal,
in his long tub,
vaguely urinous from the Victorian plumbing.
A kingly granite profile in a crimson golf-cap,
worn all day, all night,
he thinks only of his figure,
of slimming on sherbet and ginger ale —
more cut off from words than a seal.

This is the way day breaks in Bowditch Hall
   at McLean's;
the hooded night lights bring out 'Bobbie',
Porcellian '29,
a replica of Louis XVI
without the wig —
redolent and roly-poly as a sperm whale,
as he swashbuckles about in his birthday suit
and horses at chairs.

These victorious figures of bravado ossified young.

In between the limits of day,
hours and hours go by under the crew haircuts
and slighly too little nonsensical twinkle
of the Roman Catholic attendants.
(There are no Mayflower
screwballs in the Catholic Church.)

After a hearty New England breakfast,
I weigh two hundred pounds
this morning. Cock of the walk,
I strut in my turtle-necked French sailor's jersey

before the metal shaving mirrors,
and see the shaky future grow familiar
in the pinched, indigenous faces
of these thoroughbred mental cases,
twice my age and half my weight.
We are all old-timers,
each of us holds a locked razor.

Robert Lowell, from *Life Studies*

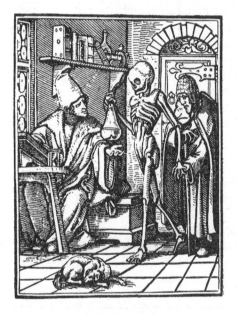

Being a patient in a foreign hospital (however efficient
that hospital), stranded and lonely and missing loved
ones, can be a trying experience. Alun Lewis and
Bernard Spencer were such patients — Lewis, during
the war, in India, and Spencer in Greece.

IN HOSPITAL: POONA

Last night I did not fight for sleep
But lay awake from midnight while the world
Turned its slow features to the moving deep
Of darkness, till I knew that you were furled,

IN HOSPITAL

Beloved, in the same dark watch as I.
And sixty degrees of longitude beside
Vanished as though a swan in ecstasy
Had spanned the distance from your sleeping side.

And like to swan or moon the whole of Wales
Glided within the parish of my care:
I saw the green tide leap on Cardigan,
Your red yacht riding like a legend there,

And the great mountains, Dafydd and Llewelyn,
Plynlimmon, Cader Idris and Eryri
Threshing the darkness back from head and fin,
And also the small nameless mining valley

Whose slopes are scratched with streets and
    sprawling graves
Dark in the lap of firwoods and great boulders
Where you lay waiting, listening to the waves —
My hot hands touched your white despondent
    shoulders

— And then ten thousand miles of daylight grew
Between us, and I heard the wild daws crake
In India's starving throat; whereat I knew
That Time upon the heart can break
But love survives the venom of the snake.

Alun Lewis, from *Ha! Ha! Among The Trumpets*, 1945

IN A FOREIGN HOSPITAL

Valleys away in the August dark the thunder
roots and tramples: lightning sharply prints
for an instant trees, hills, chimneys on the night.
We lie here in our similar rooms with the white
furniture, with our bit of Death inside us
(nearer than that Death our whole life lies under);
the man in the next room with the low voice,
the brown-skinned boy, the child among its toys
and I and others. Against my bedside light
a small green insect flings itself with a noise
tiny and regular, a 'tink; tink, tink'.

A Nun stands rustling by, saying good night,
hooded and starched and smiling with her kind
lifeless, religious eyes. 'Is there anything
you want?' — 'Sister, why yes, so many things:'
England is somewhere far away to my right
and all Your letter promised; days behind
my left hand or my head (or a whole age)
are dearer names and easier beds than here.
But since tonight must lack for all of these
I am free to keep my watch with images,
a bare white room, the World, an insect's rage,
and if I am lucky, find some link, some link.

Bernard Spencer, from Collected Poems, 1981

Lewis and Spencer were attended by compassionate and efficient medical staff. Aidan MacCarthy, an RAF doctor who was a prisoner-of-war in 1942, was not so fortunate.

I was transferred to an outside civilian hospital where a wing had been set aside for POWs. Here my elbow was X-rayed and the fractures in the bones confirmed. The Japanese surgeon who examined me seemed reasonably competent; he decided to operate the following day.

Next morning I was summoned from the ward and marched across the hospital grounds, accompanied by two armed guards. In the operating theatre, I was told to lie on the operating table, whilst my two guards stood to attention nearby. An Indonesian orderly then strapped my legs and my arms to the sides of the table. I thought this a rather odd preliminary to the anaesthetic — and then discovered there was *not* going to be any anaesthetic.

The surgeon, whom I later learned was a third-year medical student anxious to practise before going to the front, proceeded to make an incision on my elbow. I suddenly realised that he was making the cut in the wrong place. Then the blinding pain of the incision caused me to make a vain effort to break my straps. I assume I must have fainted but the pain continued. When I came to and the pain had somewhat eased off, I saw this butcher proudly holding half the head of my radius aloft in his forceps. Then he seemed to lose interest in the whole business. The Indonesian orderly took over, injected some local anaesthetic, sewed up the gaping incision, applied a dressing and gave me a sling. I was swung off the operating table and marched back to the ward. The operation seemed to have shaken even my guards. Silently they lit up cigarettes, then, mercifully, offered me one too. Shortly after my 'operation', I woke up to see my right hand and lower arm infected with a condition called erysipelas (a streptococcal infection). Normally this is a mild infection and not dangerous. But in my debilitated state, and without drugs, it was a very dangerous condition. That night an Ambonese medical orderly risked his life by stealing out over the roofs and bringing me back some sulphanilamide which he bought on the black market and which checked the infection in about three days.

Aidan MacCarthy, A Doctor's War, 1979

I am reminded of the Swiss physician Paracelsus (Bombastus) who, in the sixteenth century, listed the qualifications of a good surgeon.

A clear conscience.
Desire to learn and gather experience.
A gentle heart and a cheerful spirit.
Moral manner of life and sobriety in all things.
Greater regard for his honour than for money.
Greater interest in being useful to his patient than to himself.
He must not be married to a bigot.

Paracelsus (1493–1541)

Patients, even in ideal peacetime conditions, may not always be given a general anaesthetic for an operation. Sometimes it is necessary to undertake brain surgery

under a local anaesthetic. The patient, though conscious,
feels no pain. The operation described below took place
in Cardiff in 1938.

> Sister saying — 'Soon you'll be back in the ward,'
> sister thinking — 'Only two more on the list,'
> the patient saying — 'Thank you, I feel fine';
> small voices, small lies, nothing untoward,
> though, soon, he would blink again and again
> because of the fingers of Lambert Rogers,
> rash as a blind man's, inside his soft brain.
>
> If items of horror can make a man laugh
> then laugh at this: one hour later, the growth
> still undiscovered, ticking its own wild time;
> more brain mashed because of the probe's braille path;
> Lambert Rogers desperate, fingering still;
> his dresser thinking, 'Christ! Two more on the list,
> a cisternal puncture and a neural cyst.'
>
> Then, suddenly, the cracked record in the brain,
> a ventriloquist voice that cried, 'You sod,
> leave my soul alone, leave my soul alone,' —
> the patient's dummy lips moving to that refrain,
> the patient's eyes too wide. And, shocked,
> Lambert Rogers drawing out the probe
> with nurses, students, sister, petrified.
>
> 'Leave my soul alone, leave my soul alone,'
> that voice so arctic and that cry so odd
> had nowhere else to go — till the antique
> gramophone wound down and the words began
> to blur and slow, '. . . leave . . . my . . . soul . . .
>   alone . . .'
> to cease at last when something other died.
> And silence matched the silence under snow.

Dannie Abse, from *Collected Poems*, 1977

Finally, comes the time for the patient to go home.

He had filled out again, had a good colour and no
longer looked older than his age. Thus, to overcome

Mr E's Parkinsonism was a matter of days, but to overcome his invalidism and fear and pessimism took all of nine months. Mr E's leaving the hospital and return to his home had a moving and triumphal quality about it; half the hospital turned out to see him off, and the *New York Times* itself published a picture; it was the first time in fifty years that a Parkinsonian patient who had entered Mount Carmel had ever left it to return home.

Oliver W. Sacks, *Awakenings*, 1973

DISCHARGED FROM HOSPITAL

He stands upon the steps and fronts the morning.
The porter has called a taxi, and behind him
The infirmary doors have swung and come to rest.
Physician, surgeon and anaesthetist
Have exercised their skill and he is cured.
The rabelaisian sister with the bedpan,
The vigorous masseuse, the sensual nurse
Who washed him modestly beneath a blanket,
The dawn chorus of cleaners, the almoner,
The visiting clergyman — all proceed without him.
He is alone, beyond all need of them,
And the saved man goes home to die of health.

James Reeves, *The Questioning Tiger*

Alone in her old bedroom, her first impulse was not, after all, to tear off the clothes she had worn in the asylum. She went straight to the wardrobe glass and studied her full-length reflection. *There* she had never been able to see more than her head and shoulders. She took off the hated beige coat which had never seemed to belong to her more than the uniform brown serge dressing-gown. The old navy dress that hung so loose on the body whose thinness she approved had had its place in her real life. She felt a sudden affection for it, as if it were a loyal friend who had followed her into exile. If she could find its belt, she might even keep it on. She began to rummage through drawers in search of the scarlet belt.

She became so fascinated in discovering things she remembered and things she had forgotten she possessed that, soon, it seemed no more astonishing to be back in that room than if she had just returned from school after a particularly long and dreary term. Presently, she gave up the search for the missing belt and sat down on the bed with its faded Indian cotton bedspread. The springs sagged so violently that she realised there was not even a mattress underneath. Then she grasped that this was a very different home-coming. Perhaps they had never expected her to return at all. She pressed her knuckles to her temples trying to remember when she had last slept in that bed. What had she been doing before *it* happened? Who had taken her to Nazareth? She had a confused memory of driving somewhere in a taxi, wearing a fur coat over a nightdress. She brushed it aside. It was something *before* that she wanted to recover. Something desperately important in the real world . . . a *person*. Before she could recover this vital missing piece, her father knocked on the door:

'Nearly ready, dear?'

'Give me five minutes,' she called back.

She hurriedly changed into the first dress she pulled out of the wardrobe, went to the dressing table and combed her hair. Her brushes were still there; their silver backs tarnished. There was a bowl with a little powder and a worn puff still in it. She fluffed some powder over her face. It smelt delicious after the smell of hospital soap which still clung to her hands. The scent was not only delicious — it brought her so much nearer to what she was trying to track down that she could hardly bear to leave the bedroom to go down-stairs.

Antonia White, *Beyond the Glass*, 1954

I am out in the supermarket, choosing —
this very afternoon, this day —
picking up tomatoes, cheese, bread,

things I want and shall be using
to make myself a meal, while they
eat their stodgy suppers in bed —

Janet with her big freckled breasts,
her prim Scots voice, her one friend,
and never in hospital before,

who came in to have a few tests
and now can't see where they'll end;
and Coral in the bed by the door

who whimpered and gasped behind a screen
with nurses to and fro all night
and far too much of the day;

pallid, bewildered, nineteen.
And Mary, who will be all right
but gradually. And Alice, who may.

Whereas I stand almost intact,
giddy with freedom, not with pain.
I lift my light basket, observing

how little I needed in fact;
and move to the checkout, to the rain,
to the lights and the long street curving.

Fleur Adcock, from *The Soho Hospital for Women*,
1978

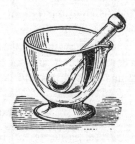

Cures

We rationalize, we dissimulate, we pretend: we pretend that Modern Medicine is a Rational Science, all facts, no nonsense, and just what it seems. But we have only to tap its glossy veneer for it to split wide open, and reveal to us its roots and foundations, its old dark heart of metaphysics, mysticism, magic and myth. Medicine is the oldest of the arts, and the oldest of the sciences: would one not expect it to spring from the deepest knowledge and feelings we have?

There is, of course, an ordinary medicine, an everyday medicine, humdrum, prosaic, a medicine for stubbed toes, quinsies, bunions and boils; but all of us entertain the idea of *another* sort of medicine, of a wholly different kind: something deeper, older, extraordinary, almost sacred, which will restore to us our lost health and wholeness, and give us a sense of perfect well-being.

For all of us have a basic, intuitive feeling that once we *were* whole and well; at ease, at peace, at home in the world; totally united with the grounds of our being; and that then we lost this primal, happy, innocent state, and fell into our present sickness and suffering. We had something of infinite beauty and preciousness — and we lost it; we spend our lives searching for what we have lost; and one day, perhaps, we will suddenly find it. And this will be the miracle, the millenium!

Oliver W. Sacks, *Awakenings*, 1973

The older, other sorts of medicine nevertheless seem strange to us today whether prescribed centuries ago in Pliny's day or now, as in some parts of Africa. I do not necessarily recommend them.

[84]

The leaves of the holly, crushed and with the addition of salt are good for diseases of the joints, while the berries are good for menstruation, coeliac trouble, dysentery and cholera. Taken in wine they check looseness of the bowels.

Pliny the Elder (23–79), *Natural History*

Remedy for guinea worms (in present day Nigeria):

If the guinea worm in your body comes out like a thread take it and put one tooth of a dead person on it. Then bind the two together with a white piece of cloth. Use this to rub your body over, nine times. Then go and bury it. You will never be attacked by it again.

Remedy for eye trouble and dizziness:

Grind many right eyes of snakes with some itiro (mascara). Apply the concoction to the eyes and you will be quickly relieved.

Una Maclean, *Magical Medicine*, 1971

These 'magical' recommendations are logical to those who believe in them. What seem to us absurd proposi- tions are so because they may be based on wrong 'medical' premises.

Some men have great glaring eyes; others again have them little and pinking. Some are goggle-eyed as if they would start out of their heads, and these are sup- posed to be dim-sighted; others are hollow-eyed, and they are thought to have the best and clearest sight, as is the case also with those which resemble in colour the eyes of the Goat. Blue eyes commonly see the clearer in the dark. It is reported of Tiberius Caesar that if he was wakened in the night, he could see everything for a while as well as in the clear day; but soon after, by little and little, the darkness would overcast everything again — a gift that no one in the world was ever known to have but himself. Augustus Caesar of famous memory had red eyes like some horses; and indeed he was wall-eyed, for the white of it was much bigger than in other men. If a man looked earnestly upon him and beheld them wistly [intently] he would be displeased and highly offended. A man could not anger him worse. Claudius Caesar had a fleshly substance about the corners of his eyes that took up a good part of the white and many times they were very red and bloodshot. Nero had a very short sight; unless he winked (as it were) and looked narrow with his eyes he could not see anything well, however near. Caligula the Emperor had twenty couples of professed sword players in his fence school and of all these only two could not be made to wink or once twinkle with their eyes, and therefore they always carried the prize and were invincible. Many men cannot choose but be evermore winking, but such are holden for fearful and timorous persons.

Eyes are the very seat and habitation of the mind and affection. From them proceed the tears of compassion. When we kiss the eye we think that we touch the very heart and soul. From hence comes our weeping; from hence gush out those streams of water that drench and run down the cheeks. But what might this water and humour be, that in hearts' grief issues in such plenty and is so ready to flow? Where may it lie at other times when we are in joy, in mirth, and repose? It cannot be denied that with the Soul we imagine, with the Mind we see, and the Eyes as vessels and instruments receiving from it that visual power and faculty send it soon after abroad. Hence it is that a deep and intentive cogitation blinds a man so that he sees nothing; namely when the sight is retired far inward. Thus it is that in the Epilepsy or Falling-sickness the eyes are open and yet see nothing: for why? The mind within is darkened.

We that are citizens of Rome have a sacred and solemn manner in use among us, to close the Eyes of those that are giving up the ghost; and when they are brought to the funeral fire to open them again. The reason of this ceremonious custom is that as it is not meet for the Eyes of a dead man to be seen by the living, so it is an equal offence to hide them from heaven, unto which this honour is due and the body now presented.

Pliny the Elder (23–79), *Natural History*

The African savages came nearer the truth; but they, too, missed it when they gathered wonderingly round one of our American travellers who, in the interior, had just come into possession of a stray copy of the New York *Commercial Advertiser* and was devouring it column by column. When he got through, they offered him a high price for the mysterious object; and being asked for what they wanted it, they said: 'For an eye medicine' — that being the only reason they could conceive of for the protracted bath which he had given his eyes upon its surface.

William James, *Selected Papers on Philosophy*

The 'best' medicine was by no means practised in the West as this interesting account by a Muslim doctor of his encounter with Christian medicine shows:

They brought to me a knight with an abscess in his leg, and a woman troubled with fever. I applied to the knight a little cataplasm; his abscess opened and took a favourable turn. As for the woman I forbade her to eat certain foods, and I lowered her temperature. I was there when a Frankish doctor arrived, who said, 'This man cannot cure them.' Then, addressing the knight, he asked, 'Which do you prefer, to live with a single leg, or to die with both legs?' 'I prefer,' replied the knight, 'to live with a single leg.' 'Then bring,' said the doctor, 'a strong knight with a sharp axe.' The doctor stretched the leg of the patient on a block of wood, and then said 'Cut off the leg with the axe, detach it with a single blow.' Under my eyes the knight gave a violent blow. He gave the unfortunate man a second blow, which caused the marrow to flow from the bone, and the patient died immediately. As for the woman, the doctor examined her and said, 'She

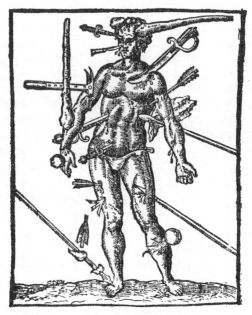

'The Wound Man', a sixteenth-century first-aid chart, showing wounds occuring during war.

is a woman with a devil in her head. Shave her hair.' They did so; she began to eat again — like her compatriots — garlic and mustard. Her fever grew worse. The doctor then said, 'The devil has gone into her head.' Seizing the razor he cut into her head in the form of a cross. Then he rubbed her head with salt. The woman expired immediately. After asking them if my services were still needed, and after receiving a negative answer, I returned, having learned from them medical matters of which I had previously been ignorant.

D. C. Munro, *Essays on the Crusades*, 1903

But a spirit of scientific enquiry was not entirely absent in the Middle Ages.

Baldwin (afterwards King of Jerusalem) had been wounded in battle while he rescued a foot soldier of his army, with whose bravery he was much delighted. The leech whom he summoned feared in his foresight lest the cataplasm outwardly applied might film over the wound, which (as he knew) had pierced deep into the prince's body; he feared therefore lest, while the skin grew smooth over the wound, it might rankle inwardly with a mass of putrid matter. This he foresaw in his wondrous skill, partly by a most praiseworthy conjecture, and partly from past experience. He therefore besought the king to command that one of the Saracen prisoners (for it would have been wicked to ask it of a Christian) should be wounded in that same place, and afterwards slain; whereby he might enquire at better leisure in the dead man's body — nay, might clearly perpend from its examination — how it was with the king's wound at the very bottom. From this however, the prince's loving-kindness shrank in horror; and he repeated that ancient example of the Emperor Constantine, who utterly refused to become the cause of any man's death, even of the basest, for so small a chance of his own safety. Then said the doctor: 'If indeed thou art resolved to take no man's life for the sake of thine own cure, then at least send for a bear, a bear that is of no use but to be baited; let him stand erect on his hinder paws with his forefeet raised, and bid them thrust him with the steel; then, by inspection of his bowels after death, I may in some degree measure how deep that wound is, and how deep thine own.' Then said the king, 'We will not strain at the beast, if need be: do therefore as thou wilt.' Whereupon it was done as the leech bade; and he discovered from this proof of the wild beast how perilous it would have been for the king if the lips of the wound had become united before the matter had been drawn forth and the bottom had grown together. Let this suffice concerning the king's pitifulness.

Quoted in G. G. Coulton, *Life in the Middle Ages*, 1929

The greatest surgeon of the sixteenth century was Ambroise Paré who effected cures where others had failed.

Having seen him, I went for a walk in a garden, and prayed God to show me this grace, that he should recover, and to bless our hands and our mendicants to cure such a complication of disease. I turned in my mind what measures I must take to this end. They called me to dinner. I came into the kitchen, and there I saw, taken out of a great pot, half a sheep, a quarter of veal, three great pieces of beef, two fowls, and a very large piece of bacon, with abundance of good herbs. Then I said to myself that the broth of the pot would be full of juices and very nourishing. After dinner, we began our conversation, all the physicians and surgeons together, in the presence of M. le Duc d'Ascot and some gentlemen who were with him. I began to say to the surgeons that I was astonished that they had not made incisions in the patient's thigh, seeing that it was all suppurating, and the thick matter in it very fetid and offensive, showing that it had long been pent-up there; and I had found with the probe caries of the bone and scales of bone already loose. They answered me, Never would he consent to it; indeed, that it was near two months since they had been able to get leave to put clean sheets on the bed, and that one scarce dared touch the coverlet, so great was his pain. Then I said, To cure him, we must touch something else than the coverlet of his bed. Each said what he thought of the malady of the patient, and in conclusion, they all held it hopeless. I told them that there was still some hope, because he was young, and God and Nature sometimes do what seems to physicians and surgeons impossible.

Paré not only treated the young man with medicines, a nourishing diet, and clean bedding, but made three open-

ings in his thigh. Slowly the patient recovered. Nor did Paré neglect the young man's convalescence.

Then, when I saw him beginning to get well, I told him that he must have viols and violins, and a buffoon to make him laugh: which he did. In a month, we got him into a chair; and he had himself carried about his garden, and to the door of his château, to watch people passing. The villagers for two or three leagues round, now that they could see him, came on holidays to sing and dance, a regular crowd of light-hearted country folk, rejoicing in his convalescence, all glad to see him, not without plenty of laughter and plenty of drink. He always gave them a hogshead of beer: and they all drank his health with a will. . . In six weeks he began to stand a little on crutches, and to put on flesh and to get a good natural colour. He wanted to go to Beaumont, his brother's place: and was taken thither in a carrying-chair, by eight men at a time. And the peasants in the villages through which we passed, when they knew it was M. le Marquis, fought who should carry him, and insisted that he should drink with them: and it was only beer but they would have given him Hippocras, if there had been any, and all were glad to see him, and prayed God for him.

Ambroise Paré, *Journeys made into Divers Places,*
1539–1569

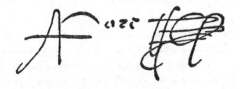

The autograph of Ambroise Paré

The spirit of scientific enquiry rarely inspired those who treated the insane. In the seventeenth century the mentally sick ceased to be the victims of priests. Instead

*they became martyrs of doctors. For almost 200 years
the medical treatment of those unfortunates consisted
of 'Reducing the Patient by Physic'.*

Over a period of eight or ten weeks the victim was
repeatedly bled, at least one pound of blood being
taken on each occasion. Once a week, or if the doctor
thought it advisable at shorter intervals, he or she was
given an emetic — a 'Brisk Vomit' as our ancestors,
with their admirable command of English, liked to call
it. The favourite Brisk Vomit was a concoction of the
roots of black hellebore. Hellebore had been used in the
treatment of the insane since the time of Melampus, a
legendary soothsayer, first mentioned by Homer. Taken
internally, the toxicologists tell us, hellebore 'occasions
ringing in the ears, vertigo, stupor, thirst, with a feeling
of suffocation, swelling of the tongue and fauces,
emesis and catharsis, slowing of the pulse and finally
collapse and death from cardiac paralysis. Inspection
after death reveals much inflammation of the stomach
and intestines, more especially the rectum.' The doses
prescribed by the old psychiatrists were too small to
be fatal, but quite large enough to produce a dangerous
syndrome, known in medical circles as 'Helleborism'.
Every administration of the drug resulted in an
iatrogenic disease of the most distressing and painful
kind. One Brisk Vomit was more than enough: there
were no volunteers for a second dose. All the later
administrations of hellebore had to be forcible. After
five or six bouts of helleborism, the time was ripe for
purgatives. Senna, rhubarb, sulphur, colocynth, anti-
mony, aloes — blended into Black Draughts or worked
up into enormous boluses, these violent cathartics
were forced, day after day, down the patient's throat.
At the end of the two-month course of bloodlettings,
vomits and purges, most psychotics were 'reduced by
physic' to a point where they were in no condition to
give trouble. These reductions were repeated every
spring during the patient's incarceration and in the

meantime he was kept on a low diet, deficient in proteins, vitamins and even calories. It is a testimony to the amazing toughness of the human species that many psychotics survived under this treatment for decades. Indeed, they did more than survive; in spite of chronic undernourishment and periodical reductions by physic, some of them still found the strength to be violent. The answer to violence was mechanical restraint and corporal punishment.

Aldous Huxley, 'Madness, Baldness, Sadness'

Insanity was an anti-social disease. But other 'anti-social illnesses' often had short shrift from doctors.

Dr Samuel Solly, president of the Royal Medical and Chirurgical Society, giving evidence to a government committee, said of syphilis that it was self-inflicted, was avoidable by refraining from sexual activity and was intended as a punishment for our sins and that we should not interfere in the matter.

News Item, 1868

We are apt to forget how different medical practice was before the Second World War. The doctor's therapeutic armoury had progressed little since the time of Hippocrates. George Orwell recounts how he was treated in a gloomy Paris hospital.

I saw on a bed nearly opposite me a small, round-shouldered, sandy-haired man sitting half naked while a doctor and a student performed some strange operation on him. First the doctor produced from his black bag a dozen small glasses like wine glasses, then the student burned a match inside each glass to exhaust the air, then the glass was popped on to the man's back or chest and the vacuum drew up a huge yellow blister. Only after some moments did I realise what they were doing to him. It was something called cupping, a treatment which you can read about in old medical textbooks but which till then I had vaguely thought of as one of those things they do to horses. . .

I watched this barbarous remedy with detachment and even a certain amount of amusement. The next moment, however, the doctor and student came across to my bed, hoisted me upright and without a word began applying the same set of glasses, which had not been sterilised in any way. A few feeble protests that I uttered got no more response than if I had been an animal. I was very much impressed by the impersonal way in which the two men started on me. I had never been in the public ward of a hospital before, and it was my first experience of doctors who handle you without speaking to you or, in a human sense, taking any notice of you. They only put on six glasses in my case, but after doing so they scarified the blisters and applied the glasses again. Each glass now drew about a dessertspoonful of dark-coloured blood. As I lay down again, humiliated, disgusted and frightened by the thing that had been done to me, I reflected that now at least they would leave me alone. But no, not a bit of it. There was another treatment coming, the mustard poultice, seemingly a matter of routine like the hot bath. Two slatternly nurses had already got the poultice ready, and they lashed it round my chest as tight as a strait-jacket while some men who were wandering about the ward in shirt and trousers began to collect round my bed with half-sympathetic grins. I learned later that watching a patient have a mustard poultice was a favourite pastime in the ward. These things are normally applied for a quarter of an hour and certainly they are funny enough if you don't happen to be the person inside. For the first five minutes the pain is severe, but you believe you can bear it. During the second five minutes this belief evaporates, but the poultice is buckled at the back and you can't get it off. This is the period the onlookers enjoy most. During the last five minutes, I noted, a sort of numbness supervenes. After the poultice has been removed, a waterproof pillow packed with ice was thrust beneath my head and I was left alone. I did not sleep, and to the best of my knowledge this was the only night of my life — I mean the only night spent in bed — in which I have not slept at all, not even a minute.

George Orwell, *How the Poor Die*

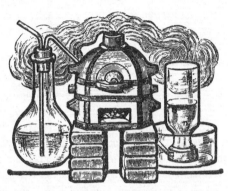

No wonder authors, earlier in this century particularly, mocked the theories and therapies of doctors.

It soon became evident that appendicitis was on its last legs, and that a new complaint had to be discovered to meet the general demand. The Faculty was up to the mark, a new disease was dumped on the market, a new word was coined, a gold coin, indeed, COLITIS!

Axel Munthe, *The Story of San Michele*, 1929

WALPOLE. I know what's the matter with you. I can see it in your complexion. I can feel it in the grip of your hand.

RIDGEON. What is it?

WALPOLE. Blood-poisoning.

RIDGEON. Blood-poisoning! Impossible.

WALPOLE. I tell you, blood-poisoning. Ninety-five per cent of the human race suffer from chronic blood-poisoning, and die of it. It's as simple as A.B.C. Your nuciform sac is full of decaying matter — undigested food and waste products — rank ptomaines. Now you take my advice, Ridgeon. Let me cut it out for you. You'll be another man afterwards.

SIR PATRICK. Don't you like him as he is?

WALPOLE. No, I don't. I don't like any man who hasn't a healthy circulation. I tell you this: in an intelligently governed country people wouldn't be allowed to go about with nuciform sacs, making themselves centres of infection. The operation ought to be compulsory: it's ten times more important than vaccination.

SIR PATRICK. Have you had your own sac removed, may I ask?

WALPOLE [*triumphantly*]. I haven't got one. Look at me! I've no symptoms. I'm as sound as a bell. About five per cent of the population haven't got any; and I'm one of the five per cent. I'll give you an instance. You know Mrs Jack Foljambe: the smart Mrs Foljambe? I operated at Easter on her sister-in-law, Lady Gorran, and found she had the biggest sac I ever saw: it held about two ounces. Well, Mrs Foljambe had the right spirit — the genuine hygienic instinct. She couldn't stand her sister-in-law being a clean, sound woman, and she simply a whited sepulchre. So she insisted on my operating on her too. And by George, sir, she hadn't any sac at all. Not a trace! Not a rudiment!! I was so taken aback — so interested, that I forgot to take the sponges out, and was stitching them up inside her when the nurse missed them.

Bernard Shaw, *The Doctor's Dilemma*, 1906

Yet it was before the Second World War that the great advances in medical therapy began — the conquest of hitherto fatal conditions such as diabetes and pernicious anaemia. And, of course, the signal discovery of such antibiotics as penicillin by Alexander Fleming, and of prontosil — the first crude sulphonamide. It is because of such advances that the doctor remains a respected figure, and the efficacy of his treatment acknowledged.

When she had left the room, the nurse told Kostoglotov to turn over on to his back again and laid sheets around the first quadrant. Then she brought up heavy mats of rubber impregnated with lead, which she used to cover all the surrounding areas which were not for the moment to receive the direct force of the X-rays. The pressure of the pliable mats, moulded to his body, was pleasantly heavy.

Then the nurse too went out and shut the door. Now she could see him only through a little window in the thick wall. A quiet humming began, the auxiliary lamps lit up, the main tube started to glow.

Through the square of skin that had been left clear on his stomach, through the layers of flesh and organs whose names their owner himself did not know, through the mass of the toad-like tumour, through the stomach and entrails, through the blood that flowed along his arteries and veins, through lymph and cells, through the spine and lesser bones and again through more layers of flesh, vessels and skin on his back, then through the hard wooden board of the couch, through the four-centimetre-thick floor-boards, through the props, through the filling beneath the boards, down, down, until they disappeared into the very stone foundations of the building or into the earth, poured the harsh X-rays, the trembling vectors of electric and magnetic fields, unimaginable to the human mind, or else the more comprehensible quanta that like shells out of guns pounded and riddled everything in their path.

And this barbarous bombardment of heavy quanta, soundless and unnoticed by the assaulted tissues, had after twelve sessions given Kostoglotov back his desire and taste for life, his appetite, even his good spirits. After the second and third bombardments he was free of the pain that had made his existence intolerable, and eager to understand how these penetrating little shells could bomb a tumour without touching the rest of the body.

Alexander Solzhenitsyn, *Cancer Ward*, 1968

I was shattered. I suppose she was the first acutely ill person I had ever seen. I thought she was dying. She was dying. She was choking, drowning in her own fluid; totally concentrating on her death. A little old lady, dank hair stuck around her head by cold sweat, every visible part moving in unison in her efforts to catch her breath. Her pale, clammy hands clutched the bars of the trolley, her eyes rolling upwards whilst her sounds were too near death to be heard. I wanted to run away. . . I had no idea what was wrong with her or what should be done. The Registrar quickly opened some vials on the side bench and injected their contents into a vein in her arm, taking a long time to do so. He fixed an oxygen mask to her nodding head, spoke a few words in a slow, unhurried way and beckoned me to follow him outside the cubicle. I accompanied him. What was it? What had he given her? Why was she dying?

'And then,' he said, leaning against the Casualty Officer's door, 'this physio comes on and does the dance of the seven veils. . .'

I was astounded. How could he stand around chatting whilst that lady lay only a few feet away? The answer was that, for him, this patient fitted into a well-known pattern. He had seen it before. He had recognised her heart failure, and treated it appropriately. Within half an hour we saw her recover enough to thank him and be wheeled off to the ward.

Lesley Isenberg in *My Medical School*, 1978

The doctor, however, sometimes errs by over-treating a patient. It has been suggested, for instance, that Hitler, through his doctor, Morell, became addicted to amphetamines or to cocaine. For my part I wish that Dr Morell had over-treated Hitler a lot more!

Linge told us that starting in late 1941 or early 1942, Hitler received an intravenous injection from Morell nearly every morning before he got out of bed. That Morell did see Hitler nearly every morning, usually before breakfast, is confirmed by the appointment book Linge kept at the time. The injection was not given because Hitler was in pain or experiencing any particular distress, but rather it was given simply as a routine part of the preparation for the day. One ampoule which was always used was labelled Vitamultin-Ca, an injectable form of the vitamin preparation manufactured at the Hamma factory. It is included in Morell's list of drugs. The critical data are supplied in descriptions of what happened when the drug was injected. Linge clearly remembers that the effects were instantly apparent — not minutes later, but while the needle was still in the arm. The effect on Hitler was obviously alerting: he felt 'fresh', alert, active, and immediately ready for the day. The purpose of the injection was obviously to energize. Linge's main point is confirmed by Russian medical authorities who stated on the basis of their intelligence that Hitler had a 'pep' injection every morning. Later in the war, probably starting in the middle of 1943, Hitler began to get injections at other times of the day. There were many witnesses to these injections and all concur as to the effects. Himmler had noted that Morell's injections made Hitler 'immediately' alert and active and both he and Dr Brandt believed that the immediacy of the alerting effect was what so impressed Hitler about Morell's injections. Traudl Junge, one of Hitler's secretaries, also told us that the effect of the injections was immediate and that Hitler became extremely alert and talkative. Assmann, too, described the effect as immediate and 'rejuvenating'. Walter Hewel, who was a representative of the foreign office on Hitler's staff and a member of Hitler's inner circle, said that Hitler called for Morell more and more often, especially when bad news came in. Hewel recalled that after the injection, Hitler became cheerful, talkative, physically active and tended to stay awake long hours into the night.

These descriptions provide critical evidence. The effects described by Linge and the other witnesses are characteristic of an injection of a stimulant drug of the amphetamine group or cocaine, and are not compatible with any other active drug.

Leonard L. Heston and Renate Heston, *The Medical Casebook of Adolf Hitler*, 1979

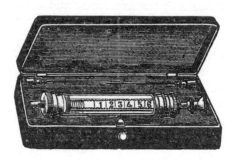

Dr Morell, no doubt, was an opportunist charlatan. But some doctors, sincere and dedicated, may be more interested in the nature of the cure than in the well-being of any single patient.

Suddenly, upon that day, the twentieth of May, nine o'clock was striking, when a sort of tall skeleton with enlarged pupils, the hollows of his cheeks touching under his palate, the torso bare, resembling a cage around which was twisted a flabby parchment, uplifted by the inhalation of a broken cough — briefly, one who was doubtfully alive, a piece of blue fox fur folded over one of his emaciated forearms, elongated the compass of his femurs in the doctor's office, while holding himself up by the large leaves of the plants.

'Tik! tik! plaff! Nothing to do!' grumbled Doctor Hallidonhill; 'am I a coroner, good for pronouncing upon the deceased? Within a week, the greater growth of this left lung will be discharged: and the right is a sieve! . . . Next!'

The attendant was about to 'remove the client', when the eminent therapeutist, slapping himself on the forehead, brusquely added, with a complex smile:

'Are you rich?'

'An arch-millionaire,' croaked, all in tears, the unfortunate personage whom Hallidonhill had just so succinctly dismissed from the planet.

'In that case, have your carriage leave you at Victoria Station! Eleven o'clock express to Dover! . . . Then the boat! . . . Then from Calais to Marseilles, sleeping car with stove! . . . And then on to Nice! There, six months of water-cress, day and night, without bread, or wine, or fruits, or meats. A spoonful of rainwater, well iodined, every other day. And water-cress, water-cress, water-cress! . . . ground, pounded in its juice . . . only chance. . . and even then! — This pretended cure with which they besiege my ears, appears to me more than absurd. I offer it to a desperate man, but without believing in it for a second. Well, everything is possible. . . Next!'

The tubercular Croesus, once delicately placed in the canopied enclosure of the elevator, the usual procession of consumptive, scorbutic, and bronchial patients began.

Six months later, the third of November, nine o'clock was striking, when a species of giant with a formidable and joyous voice, the timbre of which made the panes of glass in the office vibrate, and the leaves of the tropical plants tremble, a chubby-cheeked colossus, in rich furs, having hurled himself like a human bomb through the lamentable ranks of the clientele of Doctor Hallidonhill, penetrated without appointment-card, into the sanctum of the Prince of Science, who, cold, in his black suit, had just seated himself as usual in front of his table. Seizing his body in his arms, he lifted him like a feather, and bathing, — in silence, — the withered and sallow cheeks of the practitioner with tender tears, kissed them, and kissed them again, in a sonorous fashion, in the manner of a paradoxical Norman nurse . . . then replaced him, half in a coma, and almost suffocated, in his green armchair.

'Two millions?? Do you want them? Do you want three?' vociferated the giant, a terrible and living advertisement. 'I owe to you the breath of life, the sun, good

meals, the unbounded passions, existence, everything!
Claim, therefore, from me unheard-of remuneration! I
have a thirst for making recompense!'

'Well! really, who is this madman? . . . Have him
put out!' . . . feebly articulated the doctor after a
moment's prostration. 'But no, but no,' scolded the
giant, with the look of a boxer, which made the attendant draw back. 'In reality, I understand that you, even
you, my saviour, do not recognise me. I am the man
of the water-cress! The skeleton that was done-for, lost!
Nice! water-cress, water-cress, water-cress! . . . I have
finished my semester, and here is what you have accom-
plished. Look here; listen to this!'

And he beat upon his thorax with fists capable of
breaking the skulls of prime Middlesex bulls.

'Hein!' cried the doctor, leaping to his feet — 'you
are . . . what! This is the moribund who . . .'

'Yes, a thousand times yes, it is I!' shouted the giant:
— 'Since last evening, scarcely had I left the steamer,
when I ordered your statue in bronze, and I will know
how to have some funeral ground bestowed on you at
Westminster!'

Letting himself fall upon a vast sofa, the spring of
which creaked and groaned: '— Ah, but life is good!'
he sighed with the beatific smile of placid ecstasy.
Upon two words rapidly pronounced in a low voice by
the doctor, the secretary and the attendant withdrew.
Once alone with his resuscitated patient, Hallidonhill,
stiff, wan and icy, with a nervous eye, looked upon the
giant, during several seconds, in silence — then, all of
a sudden:

'Permit me, in the first place,' he murmured in a
strange tone, 'to remove this fly from your temple!' and
precipitating himself forward, the doctor, taking from
his pocket a short bull-dog revolver, discharged it twice,
very rapidly, into the artery of the left temple.

The giant fell, the skull fractured, bespattering with
his grateful brain, the rug of the room, which he beat
with the palms of his hands for a minute.

With ten cuts of the scissors, fur greatcoat, clothes, and under clothes, slashed at random, left bare his chest, — which the grave surgeon, with a single stroke of his large bistoury, cleft immediately from top to bottom.

A quarter of an hour later, when the constable had entered the office to beg Doctor Hallidonhill to be so good as to follow him, the latter, calm, seated before his table, his powerful magnifying glass in his hand, scrutinised a pair of enormous lungs laid out flat upon his sanguinary desk. The genius of Science was trying, in the person of this man, to find an explanation of this arch-miraculous action of the water-cress, at once lubricating and relieving.

Villiers De L'Isle-Adam, *The Heroism of
Doctor Hallidonhill*, 1883

Another kind of misplaced therapeutic enthusiasm concerned Freud's pupil Sandor Ferenczi, as can be seen from Freud's letter to him on 13 December 1931.

I see that the differences between us come to a head in a technical detail which is well worth discussing. You have not made a secret of the fact that you kiss your patients and let them kiss you; I had also heard that from a patient of my own. Now when you decide to give a full account of your technique and its results you will have to choose between two ways: either you relate this or you conceal it. The latter, as you may well think, is dishonourable. What one does in one's technique one has to defend openly. Besides, both ways soon come together. Even if you don't say so yourself it will soon get known just as I knew it before you told me.

Now I am assuredly not one of those who from prudishness or from consideration of bourgeois convention would condemn little erotic gratifications of this kind. And I am also aware that in the time of the Nibelungs a kiss was a harmless greeting granted to every guest. I am further of the opinion that analysis is possible even in Soviet Russia where so far as the State is concerned there is full sexual freedom. But that does not alter the facts that we are not living in Russia and that with us a kiss signifies a certain erotic intimacy. We have hitherto in our technique held to the conclusion that patients are to be refused erotic gratifications. You know too that where more extensive gratifications are not to be had milder caresses very easily take over their role, in love affairs, on the stage etc.

Now picture what will be the result of publishing your technique. There is no revolutionary who is not driven out of the field by a still more radical one. A number of independent thinkers in matters of technique will say to themselves: why stop at a kiss? Certainly one gets further when one adopts 'pawing' as well, which after all doesn't make a baby. And then bolder ones will come along who will go further to peeping and showing — and soon we shall have accepted in the technique of analysis the whole repertoire of demi-viergerie and petting-parties, resulting in an enormous increase of interest in psycho-analysis among both analysts and patients. The new adherent, however, will easily claim too much of this interest for himself, the younger of our colleagues will find it hard to stop at the point they originally intended, and God the Father Ferenczi gazing at the lively scene he has created will perhaps say to himself: maybe after all I should have halted in my technique of motherly affection *before* the kiss. . .

Quoted in Ernest Jones, *Sigmund Freud: Life and Work*, 1957

The happiest landscape my eyes ever meddled with —
Pines, waterfall, and a most stately lawn —
Is the view they call Paradise Pond in Northampton
at Smith.
Then comes a hedge, and a hospital further on.

CURES

My boy of three was watching me watch this view
When I learnt once more how ambiguous everything
  is.
He, too, has his dogma; he 'knows' for a fact it
  is true
That a hurt goes away at a kiss.

My eyes were so full of Paradise Pond I agreed
With my son for an instant as slim as the hedges
  that hide
'Mass. State Hospital' crammed inside
With the crazy and hurt. Is it lack of a kiss
Made the State of Mass. need a house like this?
Of course not. Or, come to think of it, yes indeed.

      Peter Viereck, from *Strike Through the Mask*, 1950

*Love certainly can be curative. This is not just a senti-
mental notion. It can be like a blood transfusion. For
that matter a blood transfusion can be sometimes like
an act of love!*

Blood Donors This Way — the notice broods
And rudely wakes my slumbering conscience
Devoted long to slaking passion's thirst;
My blood's my life and plainest common-sense
Dictates I summon all myself to fence
Away this sentimental call and quench
My better nature; but then goes in a woman
Miniskirted, beautiful as Eve.
I enter then. We lie together on the sacrificial bench
Victims to the medical profession,
And when the session's over, quench desire
In looks of mutual love while drinking tea.
Alas! We part but who knows but the fire
Of our twin blood may mingle in life-giving harmony
In some poor Lazarus little knowing why
His body teems with strange erotic alchemy.

      S. L. Henderson Smith, 'Blood Transfusion', from
                        Snow Children, 1978

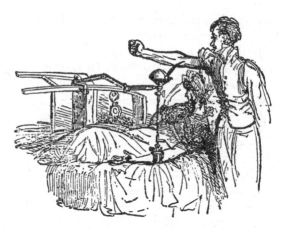

Sergeant Davis from the front office of the Hospital came in to announce that all civilian employees would have to have blood tests immediately. One of the young C.M.T.C. men had fallen out in the ninety-degree heat. The sergeant didn't know exactly what had happened to him after he had been rushed to the hospital. He had had to be operated on, had suffered a great loss of blood, and was near death. Because of Army regulations — and here the sergeant's small black eyes flickered like the balls in a pinball machine as he unwound a bit of the red tape in which he delighted — Army personnel were not allowed to give blood to civilians, and one of the civilian employees would have to be found with matching blood. Off we all went to the lab. and then right after lunch I walked home through the woods for the afternoon break as I always did. When I arrived at the house, I lay down to rest and soon the ambulance siren was closing in upon my dream, drawing closer and closer until it was right outside my door. I awoke to find it really there, outside the window. My blood type matched that of the patient, and although other employees had blood types that also matched, I was chosen as the one most readily available and the one whose absence would least disrupt hospital routine.

The ambulance rushed me back to the Hospital, and within minutes I was wheeled into the operating room, where I waited in unearthly stillness until I heard the agonising moans of the C.M.T.C. patient as he, in turn, was wheeled into the room beside me. His arm was stretched out beside mine, and when my vein was pierced and the blood pumped out and into his veins I had the sensation that the patient's groans were coming from deep within me. We were united now, this unknown young civilian in uniform, whose face I could not even see and who came probably, as many of the others did, from a farm in Missouri or southern Illinois, joined by blood, blood-brothers like the knights of the Middle Ages, united not for king or country but for the most ancient and honourable struggle of all, the struggle against death. I could hear the agony of his groaning deep within me as I was wheeled out under the slow-moving ceiling fans through the dark corridors, and I heard them still that night as I lay beside my real brother in our brass bed and prayed for him while the voices of the beer drinkers below drifted up the stairs.

William Jay Smith, *Army Brat*, 1980

It is better though to give blood than to have to receive it. Better to keep to a regimen of health such as Francis Bacon once advised. Or even, to one recommended by Dr Coué who once admonished us to say regularly 'Every day, in every way, I get better and better!'

There is a wisdom in this beyond the rules of physic: a man's own observation, what he finds good of, and what he finds hurt of, is the best physic to preserve health; but it is a safer conclusion to say, 'This agreeth not well with me, therefore I will not continue it,' than this, 'I find no offence of this, therefore I may use it:' for strength of nature in youth passeth over many excesses which are owing a man till his age. Discern of the coming on of years, and think not to

do the same things still; for age will not be defied.
Beware of sudden change in any great point of diet, and
if necessity enforce it, fit the rest to it; for it is a secret,
both in nature and state, that it is safer to change
many things than one. Examine thy customs of diet,
sleep, exercise, apparel, and the like, and try, in anything thou shalt judge hurtful, to discontinue it by
little and little; but so as if thou dost find any inconvenience by the change, thou come back to it again;
for it is hard to distinguish that which is generally
held good and wholesome, from that which is good
particularly, and fit for thine own body. To be free-
minded and cheerfully disposed at hours of meat and
sleep, and of exercise, is one of the best precepts of long
lasting.

Francis Bacon, *Of Regimen of Health*, 1597

EVERY DAY IN EVERY WAY

(Dr Coué: Every day in every way I grow better and
better)

When I got up this morning
I thought the whole thing through:
Thought, Who's the hero, the man of the day?
Christopher, it's you.

With my left arm I raised my right arm
High above my head:
Said, Christopher, you're the greatest.
Then I went back to bed.

I wrapped my arms around me,
No use counting sheep.
I counted legions of myself
Walking on the deep.

The sun blazed on the miracle,
The blue ocean smiled:
We like the way you operate,
Frankly, we like your style.

Dreamed I was in a meadow,
Angels singing hymns,
Fighting the nymphs and shepherds
Off my holy limbs.

A girl leaned out with an apple,
Said, You can taste for free.
I never touch the stuff, dear,
I'm keeping myself for me.

Dreamed I was in heaven,
God said, Over to you,
Christopher, you're the greatest!
And Oh, it's true, it's true!

I like my face in the mirror,
I like my voice when I sing.
My girl says it's just infatuation —
I know it's the real thing.

> Kit Wright, from *The Bear Looked Over the*
> *Mountain*, 1978

It is time now, alas, to conclude this small anthology —
but first I should like to raise my glass and utter an
old toast:

Here's a health to all those that we love.
Here's a health to all those that love us.
Here's a health to all those that love them
 that love those
That love them that love those that love us.

> Anonymous

Acknowledgements

The editor and publishers gratefully acknowledge permission to use copyright material in this book:

Dannie Abse: extracts from: A Poet in the Family (Hutchinson, 1974), A Strong Dose of Myself (Hutchinson, 1983); extract from 'Sister saying "Soon You'll Be Back in the Ward" . . .' from Collected Poems (Hutchinson, 1977). Reprinted by permission of Anthony Sheil Associates Ltd.

Fleur Adcock: 'I am out in the supermarket choosing', Part 4 of 'The Soho Hospital for Women', © Fleur Adcock 1979, from Selected Poems (1983). Reprinted by permission of Oxford University Press.

John Betjeman: 'Devonshire Street W1' from Collected Poems (1980). Reprinted by permission of John Murray (Publishers) Ltd.

Rhys Davies: from Print of a Hare's Foot, © 1969 Rhys Davies. Reprinted by permission of Curtis Brown Ltd., London, on behalf of the Estate of Rhys Davies.

W. H. Davies: 'The Hospital Waiting-Room' from The Complete Poems of W. H. Davies, copyright © 1963 by W. H. Davies. Reprinted by permission of Jonathan Cape Ltd., on behalf of the Executors of the W. H. Davies Estate, and of Wesleyan University Press.

Sigmund Freud: from The Life and Work of Sigmund Freud, Vol. 3, ed. Ernest Jones, © 1957 by Ernest Jones. Reprinted by permission of The Hogarth Press and of Basic Books, Inc.

Robert Gittings: extract from pp. 63–4 of John Keats (1968). Reprinted by permission of Heinemann Educational Books.

Goethe: from Autobiography, trans. John Oxenford (Sidgwick & Jackson, 1971).

Leonard L. Heston & R. Heston: from The Medical Casebook of Adolf Hitler, copyright © 1979 by L. R. and R. Heston. Reprinted by permission of William Kimber & Co., Ltd., Stein & Day Publishers, and Leonard L. Heston.

Aldous Huxley: 'Madness, Baldness, Sadness' from Collected Essays by Aldous Huxley. Copyright © 1956 by Aldous Huxley. Reprinted by permission of Mrs Laura Huxley, Chatto & Windus and Harper & Row, Publishers, Inc.

Lesley Isenberg: in My Medical School (1978), ed. Dannie Abse. Reprinted by permission of Robson Books.

Patrick Kavanagh: 'The Hospital' from Collected Poems (1972). Reprinted by permission of Mrs Kathleen Kavanagh and Martin Brian & O'Keeffe Ltd.

Alun Lewis: 'In Hospital: Poona' from Ha! Ha! Among the Trumpets. Reprinted by permission of George Allen & Unwin (Publishers) Ltd.

Robert Lowell: 'Working in the Blue' from Life Studies, copyright © 1956, 1959 by Robert Lowell. Reprinted by permission of Faber & Faber Ltd., and Farrar, Straus & Giroux, Inc.

ACKNOWLEDGEMENTS

Aidan MacCarthy: from A Doctor's War (1979). Reprinted by permission of Robson Books.

Una MacLean: from Magical Medicine (Penguin Books, 1971). Reprinted by permission of A. D. Peters & Co., Ltd.

Molière: from Le Médecin Malgré Lui, trans. George Graveley, in Six Prose Comedies of Molière (1956). Reprinted by permission of Oxford University Press.

Ogden Nash: 'Notes for the Chart in 306' from There's Always Another Windmill by Ogden Nash, copyright © 1966 by Ogden Nash. Reprinted by permission of Curtis Brown Ltd., London, and of Little, Brown & Co. First appeared in the New Yorker.

J. O'Donnell: from World Medicine, 14 November 1981. Reprinted by permission.

George Orwell: from 'How the Poor Die' in Shooting an Elephant and Other Essays by George Orwell, copyright © 1950 by Sonia Brownell Orwell; renewed 1978 by Sonia Pitt-Rivers. Reprinted by permission of A. M. Heath & Co., Ltd., the estate of the late Sonia Brownell-Orwell, Martin Secker & Warburg Ltd., and Harcourt Brace Jovanovich, Inc.

Boris Pasternak: from Doctor Zhivago (1958). Reprinted by permission of Collins Publishers.

Lord Platt: in My Medical School, ed. Dannie Abse (1978). Reprinted by permission of Robson Books.

James Reeves: 'Discharged from Hospital' from The Questioning Tiger. Reprinted by permission of William Heinemann Ltd.

Mary Remmel: from The Times, 9 June 1982. Reprinted by permission of Times Newspapers Ltd.

Oliver W. Sacks: from Awakenings (1973). Reprinted by permission of Gerald Duckworth & Co., Ltd.

Richard Selzer: from Mortal Lessons: Notes on the art of surgery, copyright © 1974, 1975, 1976 by Richard Selzer. Reprinted by permission of Chatto & Windus Ltd., and Simon & Schuster, Inc.

Bernard Shaw: from The Doctor's Dilemma. Reprinted by permission of The Society of Authors on behalf of the Bernard Shaw Estate.

Clive Sinclair: from Hearts of Gold (1979). Reprinted by permission of Allison & Busby Ltd.

S. L. Henderson Smith: 'Blood Transfusion' from Snow Children (1978). Reprinted by permission of Charles Skilton Ltd.

William Jay Smith: from Army Brat: A Memoir, copyright © 1980 by William Jay Smith. Reprinted by permission of Persea Books, Inc.

Alexander Solzhenitsyn: two extracts from Cancer Ward, trans. N. Bethell & D. Burg. English translation © The Bodley Head Ltd., 1968, 1969. Reprinted by permission of The Bodley Head Ltd., and Farrar, Straus & Giroux, Inc.

Bernard Spencer: 'In a Foreign Hospital' from Collected Poems, edited by Roger Bowen (1981), © Mrs Anne Humphreys 1981. Reprinted by permission of Oxford University Press.

Jon Stallworthy: 'A Letter from Berlin' from Root and Branch (1969). Reprinted by permission of Chatto & Windus Ltd.

John Stone: in My Medical School, ed. Dannie Abse (1978). Reprinted by permission of Robson Books.

Dylan Thomas: from Selected Letters, copyright © 1965, 1966 by The Trustees for the Copyrights of Dylan Thomas. Reprinted by permission of David Higham Associates Ltd., and of New Directions Publishing Corporation.

ACKNOWLEDGEMENTS

Lewis Thomas: from '1911 Medicine', in *The Youngest Science: Notes of a Medicine-Watcher*, copyright © 1983 by Lewis Thomas. Reprinted by permission of Viking Penguin Inc.

Patrick Trevor-Roper: in *My Medical School*, ed. Dannie Abse (1978). Reprinted by permission of Robson Books.

Peter Viereck: copyright owned by the author, Peter Viereck, from his book *Strike Through the Mask*, 1950, reprinted 1972 by Greenwood Press, 88 Post Road West, Westport, Conn. 06881.

Antonia White: from *Beyond the Glass*. Reprinted by permission of Virago Press Ltd., London.

Guy Williams: from *The Age of Agony* (1975). Reprinted by permisson of Constable & Co., Ltd.

William Carlos Williams: from *Autobiography of William Carlos Williams*, copyright © 1951 by William Carlos Williams. Reprinted by permission of New Directions Publishing Corporation.

David Wright: extract from *The Canterbury Tales* by Geoffrey Chaucer, trans. David Wright. Translation © David Wright 1984. By permission.

Kit Wright: 'Every Day in Every Way' from *The Bear Looked Over the Mountain*. Reprinted by permission of the author.

Ian Young: from *The Private Life of Islam* (Allen Lane, 1974), copyright © Ian Young 1974. Reprinted by permission of Penguin Books Ltd.

While every effort has been made to secure permission, we may have failed in a few cases to trace the copyright holder. We apologize for any apparent negligence.

Index

Abse, Dannie, 7–10, 45–6, 80
Adcock, Fleur, 82–3
Addison, Joseph, 52–4
Agbonijo, Raimi, 32–3
amputation, 11–12
anaesthesia, 45–6, 78–80
Anonymous, 109
Asclepiades, 22–3

Bacon, Francis, 107–8
Baldwin, 88–9
Barcroft, Joseph, 13
Beethoven, Ludwig van, 54–5
Bennett, Arnold, 50–1
Berlioz, Hector, 2–4
Betjeman, John, 61–2
blood, 105–7
body-snatching, 4
Burke and Hare, 4
Buzzati, Dino, 74

Carlill, Hildred, 14
Chaucer, Geoffrey, 23–4
Chekhov, Anton, 71–2
cocaine, 98–100
colitis, 95
Coulton, G. G., 88–9
cremation, 30–2
cupping, 93–4

Davies, Rhys, 30–2
Davies, W. H., 44–5
Dickens, Charles, 69–70
dissection, 1–4, 6–9

Evelyn, John, 66–7
eyes, 85–7

Ferenczi, Sandor, 103–4
Fielding, Henry, 24–7
Freud, Sigmund, 103–4

Gittings, Robert, 10–11

Goethe, J. W. von, 57–8
Graham, James, 27–9

'Hallidonhill, Dr', 100–3
Hellebore, 92–3
Henderson Smith, S. L., 105
Hertzler, Arthur E., 37
Heston, L. L. and R., 98–100
Hippocrates, 17, 18–19
Hitler, Adolf, 98–100
Holmes, Oliver Wendell, 18–19
Hood, Thomas, 4–5
Huxley, Aldous, 92–3
hypochondria, 51–4

insanity, 91–3
Isenberg, Lesley, 98

James, William, 87
Jameson, Eric, 27–9
Johnson, Samuel, 55–7
Jones, Ernest, 103–4
Juettner, Otto, 12–13

Kavanagh, Patrick, 66
Keats, John, 10–11
Kisfaludi, Karoly, 49–50
Kostov, Dr, 34–7

Lamb, Charles, 63–4
Lewis, Alun, 76–7
lithotomy, 67
Livingstone, R., 17
Lloyd George, David, 29
Lowell, Robert, 74–6
Lucas, Billy, 10–11

MacCallan, A. F., 13
MacCarthy, Aidan, 78–9
Maclean, Una, 33, 85
Molière, 39–40, 52
Morell, Dr, 98–9

Munro, D. C., 88
Munthe, Axel 95

Nash, Ogden, 65–6

O'Donnell, J., 61
Orwell, George, 93–5
Osler, Sir William, 37–8, 42

Paracelsus, 79
Paré, Ambroise, 90–1
Pasternak, Boris, 1–2
Plato, 19–21
Platt, Lord, 6–7, 13
Pliny the Elder, 21–3, 85–7
Price, Dr William, 30–2
Prior, Matthew, 37

quacks, 27–9

Rabelais, François, 59–60
Reeves, James, 81
Remmel, Mary, 46–8

Sacks, Oliver W., 62, 80–1, 84
Selzer, Richard, 5–6, 71
Semple, James G., 27
Shaw, Bernard, 95–6
Sinclair, Clive, 51–2
Singer, Charles, 19
Smith, William J., 106–7
Smollett, Tobias, 15–16

Solly, Samuel, 93
Solzhenitsyn, Alexander, 62–3, 97
Spencer, Bernard, 77–8
Stallworthy, Jon, 40–2
Stone, John, 43
Swift, Jonathan, 38–9
syphilis, 93

Thomas, Dylan, 58–9
Thomas, Lewis, 37–8
Trevor-Roper, Patrick, 13–15
Turgenev, Ivan, 29–30
typhoid, 37–8

Vesalius, 5–6
Viereck, Peter, 104–5
Villiers de l'Isle-Adam, comte de, 100–3

Warren, J. Collins, 11–12
White, Antonia, 81–2
Williams, Guy, 68–9
Williams, William Carlos, 43
Woodward, Sir Stanley, 13–14
Wright, Kit, 108–9

X-rays, 97

Young, Ian, 34–7